The Pregnant Patient

OrangeBooks Publication

1st Floor, Rajhans Arcade, Mall Road, Kohka, Bhilai, Chhattisgarh 490020

Website: **www.orangebooks.in**

First Edition, 2026

ISBN: 978-93-7426-131-6

Price: Rs. 500.00

Printed in India

THE PREGNANT PATIENT

A COMPREHENSIVE ORAL CARE GUIDE

DR. SAHRISH TARIQ

OrangeBooks Publication
www.orangebooks.in

Introduction

Many physiological changes can be seen in a female body[1] during the course of pregnancy, (which is the period in which the fetus develops in the womb) along with various changes in the oral cavity. For a normal progression of pregnancy,[2] there is an increase in the secretion of the female sex hormones, the estrogen level increases by 10 times whereas progesterone levels increase 30 times. Due to such an increase in the hormone levels along with the fetal growth, many local as well as systemic physiological and physical changes can be seen in a woman. It is a dynamic physiological state which is proved by many transient changes. These changes can develop as varied physical signs and symptoms that may have an effect on the patient's health, perceptions, and interactions with others within the surroundings. A pregnant woman requires medical monitoring or intervention, preventive care, and physical and emotional assistance during this gestation period. The systems that show major systemic changes are as follows:

- Cardiovascular systems
- Hematologic systems
- Respiratory systems
- Renal systems
- Gastrointestinal systems
- Endocrine systems
- Genitourinary systems

Due to this sudden increase in the hormone level during pregnancy, many changes are noted in the mother's body and the oral cavity is no exception.[3]

Gingival and periodontal diseases are more susceptible in pregnant women due to the biochemical and hormonal changes. Also, it is reported that different oral lesions are common during pregnancy. It has also been documented that there is an increased prevalence of dental alterations particularly caries and erosions[4] in a woman during her pregnancy. Since the old wives' tale of "the loss of a tooth for every pregnancy," oral health during pregnancy has long been a focus of interest.[5]

Patients, physicians, and dentists usually avoid treatment of oral health problems throughout physiological conditions. This drawback is attended by lack of clinical pointers for the management of common oral conditions throughout physiological conditions. In the absence of practice guidelines, fear of medico-legal action based on the negligent or substandard treatment of oral conditions during pregnancy abounds, however it is largely unfounded.[6] Keeping aside the lack of practice standards there are more barriers to dental care during pregnancy which include the following:

a) Inadequate dental insurance

b) Persistent myths about the effects of pregnancy on dental health

c) Concerns for foetal safety during dental treatment.[7]

Therefore, it is essential for the management of the pregnant and nursing mothers[8] to understand the physiologic changes of the body and the effects of dental radiation, and the medications which are used in dentistry for pregnant women, lactating mothers and fetuses.

Physiology of Pregnancy and Treatment Consideration

It is seen that during pregnancy, the normal physiologic mechanisms which are responsible for maintaining homeostasis undergo noticeable changes. Specifically, systemic alterations in cardiovascular, respiratory, and hematologic systems should be carefully monitored by the surgeon. Gastrointestinal, renal, and endocrine alterations are also important to mention as they may require modifications of treatment protocols.

Contents

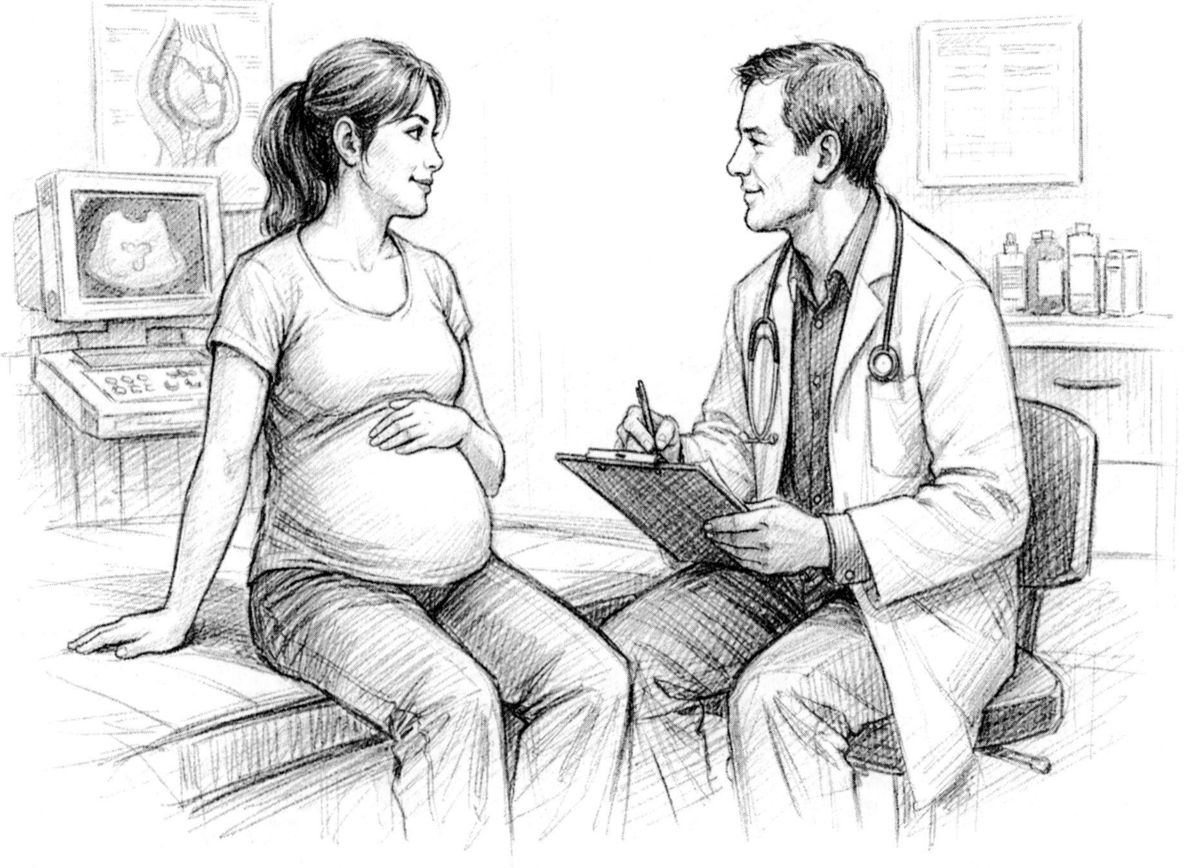

Pregnancy and Health

Physiology

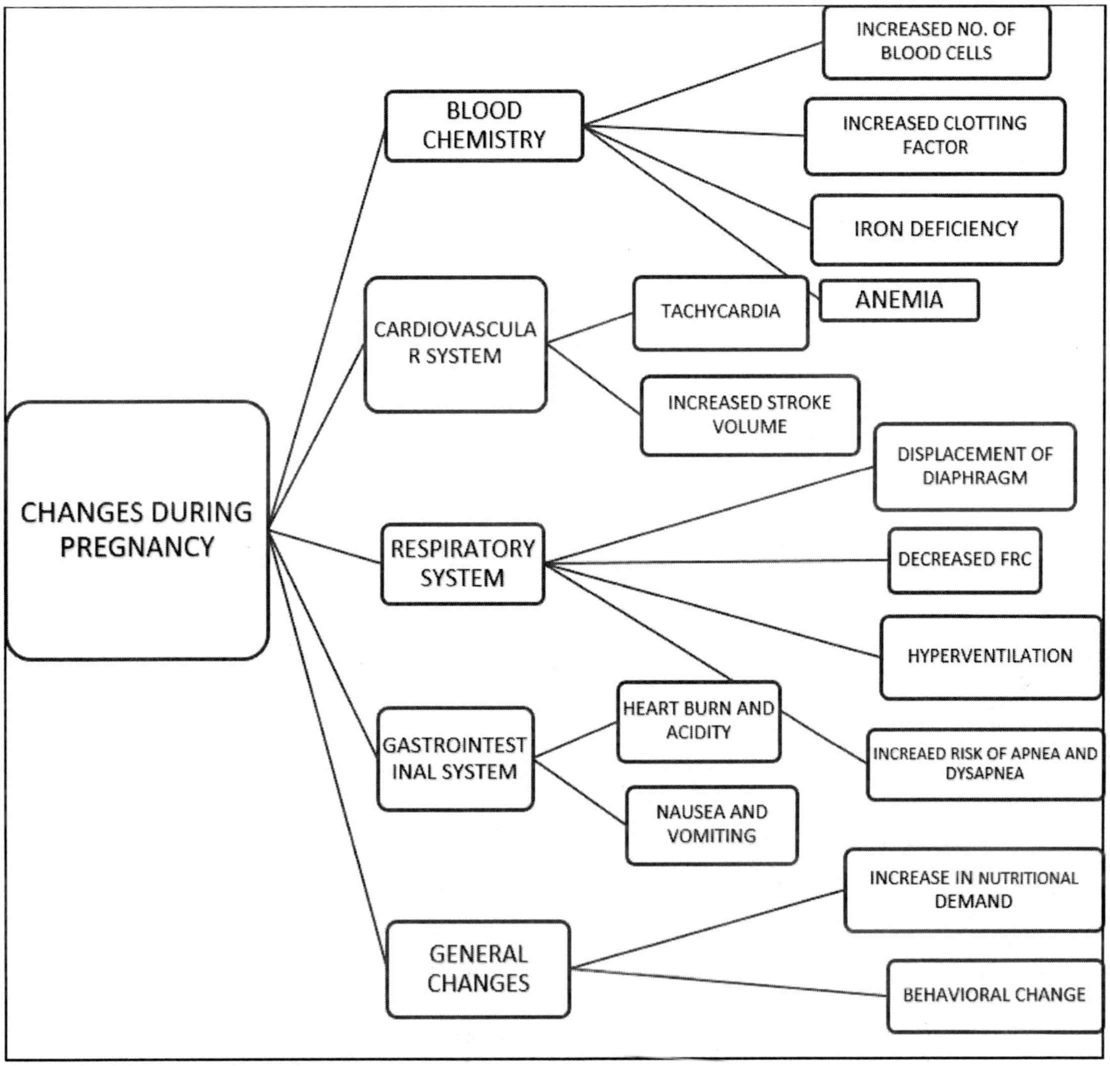

I. Cardiovascular Alterations

In comparison to the females who are not pregnant, the pregnant patient shows significant changes in blood volume and cardiac output i.e. the heart rate and stroke volume, and also changes in systemic vascular resistance and blood pressure.[8,9-15] It has been seen that in the pregnant patient the total blood volume can increase by up to 50% by 32 weeks gestation. This rise can be primarily attributed to a rise in plasma volume and secondary anemia.[8,14,15] Primarily due to increase in the stroke volume and secondarily due to the increase in heart rate.[8,10,16-18] an increase in cardiac output is apparent in the third trimester i.e. gestational weeks 25–33. It is clinically evident that in 90% of pregnant patients[17] there is an increase in cardiac output accompanied by functional S3 systolic murmur. The blood pressure drastically decreases to the baseline levels by the end of the second trimester[19] in contrast to changes in cardiac output. Due to a decrease in the systemic vascular resistance, there is a decrease in systolic and diastolic blood pressure early in pregnancy which is the lowest levels during weeks 16 and 24 although the mechanism of this decrease is not well established.[11,12] There are many mediators indicated by current data eg, progesterone, prostaglandins, and nitric oxide as causing peripheral vasodilation and venodilation.[13,15,16]

1. Hypertension (Increased Blood Pressure)

It has been seen that in about 7% to 10% of pregnancies[20,21] hypertensive disorders occur. If a woman is experiencing hypertension before the 20th week of pregnancy[8,20] this condition is known as Pre-existing hypertension. Following are the two indications of pre-existing hypertension:

a) a systolic blood pressure ≥ 140 mmHg

b) a diastolic blood pressure≥ 90 mmHg.

If a woman becomes hypertensive for the first time during the second half of pregnancy[20] this condition is well known as Pregnancy-induced hypertension. This pregnancy-induced hypertension is indicated by:

a) systolic blood pressure ≥ 30 mmHg

b) diastolic blood pressure ≥ 15 mmHg

2. Pre-eclampsia

Usually, after week 20 of pregnancy[20-23] it has been seen that in about 3% to 7% of women, pre-eclampsia occurs. It can be caused or preceded by liver dysfunction.[8] Periodontal disease has been found to be associated with pre-eclampsia in pregnant women.[22]

Factors in Diagnosis Include the Following[44-47]

Hypertension, Including Pregnancy-induced Hypertension (blood pressure above 140/90 mmHg on two readings that are at least 4 hours apart), Proteinuria, Edema. Still, the exact cause is not known.

Family or personal history of pre-eclampsia·, age (younger than 20 or older than 35 years)· Primigravida (pregnant for the first time), Diabetes, Pre-existing hypertension, or pre-existing vascular disorders.[22,] High pre-pregnancy blood pressure or weight (the higher these values, the higher the risk for pre-eclampsia) are some of the predisposing factors.

Risk factors include:

- Multiple gestation, that includes twins or triplets
- Change in paternity from the previous pregnancy
- Different parental ethnicity

Blood pressure > 160/108, Pulmonary edema, Less than 5 g proteinuria over a 24-hour period, and there is an increased risk of fetal intrauterine growth restriction or IUGR are associated with severe pre-eclampsia.

Placental abruption, where the placenta separates from the inner uterine wall prior to delivery, HELLP syndrome (hemolysis, elevated liver enzymes, and low platelet count), and Pre-eclampsia may progress to eclampsia are some life-threatening complications that come along with pre-eclampsia.

Delivery is the only cure for pre-eclampsia.

3. Eclampsia

Eclampsia includes convulsive seizures or coma that does not have another etiology and occur during pre-eclampsia.[20,21] More than 80% of women with eclampsia are young women who are pregnant for the first time (primigravida).

The pathogenesis includes the following:

- Uterine spiral arteries, which supply nutrients to the placenta and fetus, do not dilate. This decreases placental perfusion.
- Increased maternal vasopressor sensitivity.
- Coagulation cascade activation with concomitant micro-thrombi.
- Decreased intravascular volume.

There is an increased risk of Cerebral hemorrhage, Aspiration pneumonia, Hypoxia, Encephalopathy, Thromboembolism, Poor perinatal outcome (diabetic patients), and Maternal and/or fetal death (Maternal death is often due to gastric aspiration, and fetal death is often due to hypoxia)

Eclamptic seizures are considered to be a medical emergency if 25% occur before labor or 50% occur during labor or 25% occur 7 to 10 days postpartum.

Treatment of eclampsia may include:

- Delivery (best treatment)
- Medication for seizure prophylaxis
- Medication to control blood pressure
- Anti-platelet therapy (including aspirin and heparin)
- Calcium supplements

When the pregnant patient is placed in a supine position due to increased abdomino-pelvic mass there are chances that there is significant compression of the inferior vena cava by the fetus. There is a decrease in stroke volume and a compensatory baroreceptor reflex in order to maintain cardiac output, which is the result of compression. The supine hypotension syndrome is clinically characterized by the following:

- Hypotension
- Syncope
- Bradycardia

Even if the patient is not showing the symptoms of supine hypotension syndrome, there is a potential for significant disruption of utero placental flow when the patient is supine. Following is the way to prevent or alleviate supine hypotension: the pregnant patients should be rolled to the left side by 5° to 15° it is a position in which the right hip is elevated 10–12 cm.[20,24,25] This can be achieved by inserting a wedge or pillow under the right hip. In case this does not work to alleviate the hypotension, the patient can be placed in a full left lateral position.

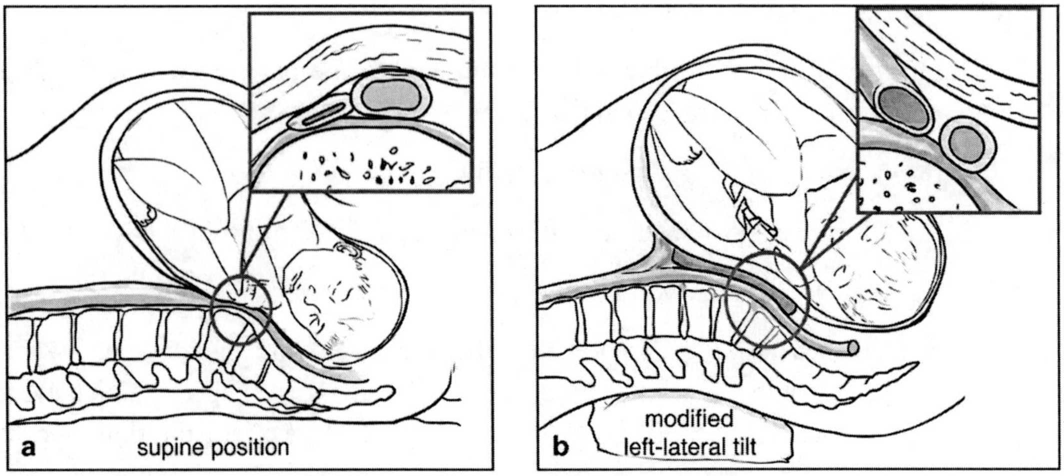

A statement was published by the California Dental Association in 2010 which which states that pre-eclampsia is not a contraindication to dental care. However, patients with pre-eclampsia often have higher blood pressure, which should be monitored closely.

A statement was published by the California Dental Association in 2010 published which state that pre-eclampsia is not a contraindication to dental care. However, patients with pre-eclampsia may be taking certain medications and may therefore require additional consideration when providing dental treatment. Physicians may treat some subgroups with aspirin, anti-platelet agents, calcium, and heparin.[22] Other treatment options include anti-hypertensives, corticosteroids, or anticonvulsant medications.[10] Prior to any dental procedures it should be ensured that all the patients provide a complete list of prescription and over-the-counter medicines. A patient with pre-eclampsia or eclampsia may be at increased risk of seizure when lidocaine is accidentally administered intravascularly.[21] Consider consulting with the patient's prenatal care provider when pre-eclampsia is either present or suspected.

Eclamptic seizures are considered a medical emergency.[20] Most eclamptic seizures (75%) occur in the time frame from labor to 10 days postpartum.The risk of an eclamptic seizure occurring during dental treatment can be reduced by deferring elective dental treatment during this time frame. It should be kept in mind that the patient's medical provider could have prescribed medication that could lead to interference with dental treatment. Following is an example: antiplatelet therapy ie. Use of, aspirin or heparin may increase bleeding risk during surgery.

4. Cardiopulmonary Arrest

It is noted that out of 12,000[26] pregnancies only 1 patient has shown an incidence of cardiac arrest during pregnancy. During a respiratory arrest in pregnant patients anoxia can rapidly occur due to respiratory changes and decreased ability to buffer pH to compensate for respiratory problems. Fetus has several protective measures during severe hypoxia. By increasing blood flow the to the placenta the fetal cardiac output is altered so as to increase the gaseous exchange. In order to protect the vital organs from severe damage the fetal blood is redirected towards. The fetal hemoglobin has a higher tendency to bind with oxygen than maternal haemoglobin as fetal red blood cells (RBCs) contain more fetal hemoglobin than maternal haemoglobin.[27] Few modifications to cardiopulmonary resuscitation has been recommended by The American Heart association (AHA). During pregnancy Automated external defibrillators (AEDs) can be used without any modification.[26] It is recommended to provide supplemental oxygen to the pregnant patients as they have increased oxygen demand because of the fetus. As the pregnancy progresses, aortocaval compression can occur by the gravid uterus, preventing adequate return circulation during CPR.[26,27] In case the aortocaval compression is present during CPR,[28,29] it is likely that the resuscitation attempts will fail. In order to address this problem of aortocaval compression the woman's body can be tilted towards her left side. But the problem that one might face is that if the woman's body is tilted, her heart can shift laterally, which can in turn decrease the effectiveness of chest compression hence, resulting in a non successful resuscitation.[26] In order to position a pregnant women into

Left Uterine Displacement (LUD) during a dental treatment, the dental provider may place a pillow or a wedge under the woman. It should also be kept in mind that pillows or wedges tend to slip during CPR.[28] In order to relieve aortocaval compression, continuous manual LUD (which is the preferred can be done by having someone either pull or push the gravid uterus· One should avoid pressing down on the woman..

Manual LUD should be done under the following circumstances[26]:

- Gestational age at least 20 weeks
- Uterus is palpated at or above the umbilicus
- Difficult to assess the uterus (eg, morbidly obese patients)

Emergency cesarean delivery may be required· Arrange emergency transportation that can handle both the patient and the fetus.[27] If the patient recovers, position her in the full left lateral decubitus position if possible until emergency medical services (EMS) arrive to transport her to a hospital.[26]

II. Respiratory Alterations

Due to increased oxygen demands of the maternal-fetal systems changes can be seen in respiratory physiology.There are notable increases in tidal volume and minute ventilation rate, which are caused by the superior displacement of the diaphragm.[8,9,19,30,31] There is a rise in intrathoracic pressure due to this displacement which can be up to 3 cm - 4 cm,which leads to an increase in the anteroposterior diameter of the thorax and chest circumference during inspiration.[8] In addition to the increase in ventilation, there is a concomitant decrease in oxygen reserve and an increase in oxygen demand. Decreases in the oxygen reserves are significant because they predispose the mother and fetus to hypoxia.[8,16,17] Although hypercapnia is not a typical physiologic change in pregnant women, dyspnea is a relatively common occurrence.[8,30, 31] Up to 50% of patients exhibit this clinical sign by the middle of the second trimester, and up to 75% exhibit it by the middle of the third trimester.[30]

Hyperventilation is also a common finding in pregnant patients and is present in approximately 40% of patients late in pregnancy.[8,32] There are significant mucosal changes in the upper airways along with changes in pulmonary physiology. Upper airways mucosa has a propensity to become friable and edematous. Up to one-third of pregnant women experience severe rhinitis, which predisposes them to frequent nosebleeds and upper respiratory tract infections.[8] It has been suggested that increased serum estrogen concentrations contribute to the episodes of rhinitis seen in pregnant women.[8,33,]

Because of the effects of hyperventilation, a pregnant patient can present with a mild respiratory alkalosis.[34] Research suggests that 25% of pregnant some patients develop an abnormal alveolar-arterial oxygen gradient and some show the symptoms of moderate hypoxemia when placed in the supine position.[35] Ventilation patterns and patient position must be adjusted for the pregnant patient so as to avoid hypoxemia.[36]

III. Hematologic Alterations

Following are the hematologic changes in the gravid patient:

1. Increase in the number of erythrocytes and leukocytes
2. Increase in erythrocyte sedimentation rate
3. Increase in most of the clotting factors

These changes causes a hypercoagulable state.[8,17,37,38] A relative decrease in blood hemoglobin concentration[8,17]can also be seen. The increase in the volume of the plasma exceeds that of the erythrocyte, that leads to a physiologic anemia.[8,9] The leukocytosis that is seen in pregnancy[8,37] is attributed to increased levels of circulating catecholamines and cortisol.

A pregnant women is at an increased risk for thromboembolic events[8,9] due to a relative increase in many of the clotting factors (VII–X) and a decrease in anticlotting factors (XI, XIII). It has been reported that pregnant women have a fivefold increase in the likelihood of thromboembolic events, compared with non pregnant patients.[9,39] The hypercoagulable state and compression of venous return from the lower extremity by the uterus cause an increased risk which in turn results in venous stasis and predisposes patients to thrombus formation.[9] It has been calculated that approximately 0.10% of pregnant patients have thrombus formation; and approximately 20% of these women develop a pulmonary embolism, with a mortality rate[9,40,41] of 12% to 15% Anticoagulant therapy is the treatment of choice for a pregnant patient with a confirmed thromboembolic event or deep venous thrombosis or pulmonary embolism. For pregnant patients with a history of thromboembolic disease, it is recommended Anticoagulant prophylaxis. For such patients, Low molecular weight heparin is preferred over Coumadin for such patients as it does not cross the placenta, and has a much more predictable dose-response due to the fact that it has low protein-binding unlike unfractionated heparin, and has been demonstrated to be more effective than heparin for prophylaxis and less likely to cause major spontaneous bleeding.[9,42,43]

Antiphospholipid Syndrome

APLS also known as Antiphospholipid syndromeis a disease where antiphospholipid antibodies bind to phospholipids and this might cause thrombosis and fetal loss. During pregnancy, women with APLS are at significant risk for thromboembolism. They may be placed on anticoagulant therapy to prevent thrombus formation.[44] Because APLS carries an increased risk of thromboembolism and likelihood of increased bleeding, it is recommended to provide dental care to these patients in a hospital setting.[9]

IV. Gastrointestinal Alterations

The following are the most prominent gastrointestinal changes that occur in the gravid patient:

- Changes in intragastric pressure
- Hormonal changes
- Alterations in hepatic function.

Gastrointestinal changes:

Following are the gastrointestinal changes:

a) Increased frequency of nausea/vomiting.

b) Episodes of pyrosis (heartburn).

Approximately two-thirds of pregnant patients complain of nausea and vomiting, with the peak frequency at the end of the first trimester.[9,45] Excessive vomiting has been reported to occur in less than 1% of all pregnancies.[45] Pyrosis has been reported to occur in up to 70% of pregnant women and is thought to be the result of an increase in the intragastric pressure (caused by the presence of the fetus) and concomitant decreases in smooth muscle tone of the lower esophageal sphincter.[9,46] It is thought that the inhibition of motilin production which is caused due to high levels of progesterone is the cause of loss of lower esophageal sphincter tone. In addition to contributing to pyrosis, loss of lower esophageal sphincter tone and increased intragastric pressure have been linked to the slowing of gastric emptying rates.[9,47] Alterations in hepatic function include decreases in total protein and albumin levels and increases in serum alkaline phosphatase, cholesterol, triglyceride, bilirubin, and aminotransferase (AST, ALT) levels.[18,48,49] The reported frequency of abnormal liver function tests as a result of pregnancy is approximately 3%.[48]

For the pregnant patient with frequent or excessive vomiting, morning appointments should not be scheduled.[8] It is advised to the patient to avoid foods that could initiate nausea/ vomiting, mostly fatty foods. Dehydration and electrolyte imbalances can be seen in the patients that witness frequent episodes of vomiting. Patients with frequent vomiting should be encouraged to drink electrolyte-rich fluids, such as commercially available sports drinks.[50,51] Increased episodes of gastric reflux and regurgitation warrant special consideration because they can lead to aspiration of gastric contents and, in some cases, death.[9,52]

Keeping aside the fact that there is currently no evidence to supports the theory that antacids or histamine antagonists can be used to reduce mortality from aspiration,[53-57] it has been verified that the acidity of the gastric aspirate is directly related with mortality. Keeping this in mind the major focus of the practitioner should be to prevent the aspiration of gastric contents during surgery. Peripheral edema caused by loss of oncotic pressure can be caused due to changes in the serum concentration of liver proteins, particularly albumin. Extremity edema should be carefully monitored before and during treatment of the pregnant patient which can be caused due to concomitant hemodynamic changes in blood pressure.

V. Renal alterations

The pregnant patient typically shows the following:

- Increase in renal plasma flow
- Increase in glomerular filtration rate
- A slight decreased serum creatinine levels
- Decrease in blood urea nitrogen.

Pregnant patients have a greater risk of urinary tract infections[8,9,15,48,59] as they urinate more frequently. There is an increase in renal plasma flow primarily and decreases thereafter,during the second trimester this is caused due to increases in blood volume and peak at 60% to 80% above normal levels. In the first trimester,there is a concomitant increase in glomerular filtration rate by 30% to 50% and remains at these levels until term.[9,60] A decline in serum creatinine and blood urea nitrogen is seen due to the following:

- Increase in the filtration
- Clearance of creatinine
- Increase in uric acid, and urea

A pregnant patient should be asked to urinate before starting treatment due to the reason that they have an increased frequency of urination than normally seen. If kept untreated[9,61,62] asymptomatic bacteriuria in the pregnant patient can progress to urinary tract infection which can then lead to pyelonephritis. The surgeon should evaluate the patient for potential risk factors for asymptomatic bacteriuria before placing urinary catheters in a pregnant patient, which are as follows:

- Age of parity
- Sexual activity
- Presence of sickle cell trait

- Low socioeconomic status.

Because of should have their The doses of any medications that are cleared by renal excretion should be adjusted according to account for increased clearance rates[9,62] due to alterations in renal plasma flow and glomerular filtration rate.

VI. Endocrine Changes

The placenta secretes the following female sex hormones which are responsible for most of the physiological changes that occur during pregnancy:

a) Estrogen

b) Progesterone

c) Human gonadotrophin.

Thyroxine, steroids, and insulin levels are also elevated. There is an increase in the size of the thyroid gland up to 50%. There is an increase in serum thyroid-binding globulin and thyroxine due to the placental secretion of human chorionic thyrotropin (a specific thyroid-stimulating hormone).[60] There is an increase in the circulating 1,25, dihydroxy-cholecalciferol (vitamin D) levels due to an increase in circulating serum parathyroid hormone levels by up to 50%. Corticosteroid levels are increased moderately. There is a 2-fold increase in aldosterone and a 3-fold increase in cortisol levels.[9] Since Estrogen and progesterone are insulin adversaries, the increased levels of these hormones lead to insulin resistance, and in order to compensate for this resistance, the insulin levels in pregnant women are elevated. Gestational diabetes is more prevalent in obese women and in women with a positive family history of type II diabetes and about 45% of pregnant women develop gestational diabetes due to the reason that they are unable to produce sufficient amounts of insulin to overcome the action of estrogen and progesterone.

VII. Oral and Facial Changes

Following are some oral changes that are seen in pregnancy:

a) Gingivitis

b) Gingival Hyperplasia

c) Pyogenic Granuloma

d) Salivarychanges.

e) Increased Facial Pigmentation.

Pregnant women is predisposed to gingivitis and gingival hyperplasia[63] as a result of increased capillary permeability which is caused due to elevated circulating estrogen. Pregnancy gingivitis usually affects marginal and interdental papilla and is related to preexisting gingivitis. oral changes caused by hormones can be prevented or their severity can be reduced by adopting good oral hygiene.

If a patient has a pre-existing periodontal condition, pregnancy can worsen it but will not cause any such condition. Pyogenic granuloma or pregnancy tumor occurs in about 1% to 5% of pregnant women.[64] Pyogenic granuloma[65] is believed to be caused due to increased angiogenesis which is caused due to sex hormones coupled with gingival irritation by local factors such as plaque. Labial aspect of the inter-dental papilla is mainly susceptible to this. It can happen at any time during pregnancy, but is reported to be most common in first pregnancies, during the first and the second trimesters, and may regress after the child's birth.[66]

Erosion of teeth on lingual and palatal surfaces of incisors has been mentioned in a case report, but to our knowledge, there is no clinical study available to support this finding.[67,50] Salivary changes in pregnancy involve the following:

- Its Flow
- Composition
- PH
- Hormone Levels.

a) **Cross-sectional studies show the following:** a reduced whole stimulated salivary flow rate in pregnant women.

b) **Longitudinal studies show the following:** there is no change in the whole stimulated salivary flow rate.

Following are the changes that are seen in the composition of the saliva:

- A decrease in sodium
- Decrease pH
- Increase in potassium
- Increase in protein
- Increase in estrogen levels.

Physiologic Changes in Pregnancy

In order to detect the risk potential for preterm labor[68] salivary estrogen level has been suggested as a screening test. Women destined to have normal term deliveries have lower 'salivary estrogen than in women who are destined to have preterm pregnancies Salivary estrogen also increases the proliferation and desquamation of the oral mucosa increases subgingival crevicular fluid levels. The desquamating cells provide a suitable environment for bacterial growth by providing nutrition predisposing pregnant women to dental caries.[69]

There is an increase in facial pigmentation called melasma or the ''mask of pregnancy," appearing as Bilateral brown patches in the mid-face appear as facial pigmentation called melasma also known as "the mask of pregnancy." During the first trimester, these facial changes start to begin and are seen in up to 73% of pregnant women. The etiology of this condition is unknown but is believed to be related to the increase in serum estrogen and progesterone. Melasma usually resolves after parturition.[70]

A link between periodontal disease and preterm low birth weight has been suggested in recent studies. Lopez et al, in an investigation of 400 women who had gingivitis and periodontal disease, found a positive correlation between periodontal disease and low birth weight. The periodontal disease seemed to be an independent risk factor for birth weight and was decreased by good oral hygiene and periodontal treatment. There has been found a casual explanation about the positive correlation between periodontal diseases and low birth weight in several animals and human case-control studies.[71]

S.n.	System	Non-Pregnant Patient	Pregnant Patient	Direction of Change	Special Considerations
1	Cardiovascular Blood Volume (L)	4.5 -5.0	6.2- 6.7	↑	Increased Uterine mass → compression of IVC → venous stasis and increased risk for deep venous thrombosis
2	Heart rate (beats/min)	70 ± 10	80 ± 10	↑	Decreased amplitude of T-waves on electrocardiogram
3	Cardiac output (L/min)	4.3 ± 0.90	6.2 ± 1.0	↑	Extra heart sounds →systolicS3 murmur
4	Systemic vascular resistance (dyne/cm/sec)	1530 ±520	1210 ±266	↓	
5	Systolic blood pressure (mmHg)	120	110(trimester 1-2)	↓	
6	Diastolic blood pressure (mmHg)	80	50– 60 (trimester 1- 2)	↓	
7	Pulmonary Tidal volume (mL)	500	700	↑	Increased mucosal fragility →increased risk of airway edema, epistaxis with manipulation of nasal airway
8	Minute ventilation (L)	7	10	↑	Decreased PaO_2 while

					supine→increased risk of hypoxia. decreased functional residual capacity, progesterone-induced hyperventilation
9	Hematologic Erythrocyte count (cells/mm^3)	$4\text{-}5 \times 10^5$	$4.8\text{-}6.5\times 10^5$	↑	The hypercoagulable state →increased risk for thrombosis/ embolism
10	Leukocyte count (cells/mm^3)	$5\text{-}9\times 10^3$	$5\text{-}12\times 10^3$	↑	Leukocytosis
11	Serum hemoglobin (g/100ml)	12-16	11.5-12.3	↑	Physiologic anemia due to increased circulating volume
12	Erythrocyte sedimentation rate (mm/h)	0-20	0-20	No change	Generalized immunosuppression
13	Gastrointestinal/hepatic total protein (g/dL)	6.5-7.5	5.7-6.5	↓	Loss of lower esophageal sphincter tone →increased risk of reflux disease
14	Albumin (mg/dL)	3.2-3.8	2.4-3.1	↓	Decreased gastric mobility
15	Alkaline Phosphate (IU/L)	30-115	100-120	↑	Increased intragastric pressure
16	Aspartate aminotransferase (IU/L)	0-42	› 72	↑	Loss of intravascular protein →decreased oncotic pressure→peripheral edema

17	Alanine aminotransferase (IU/L)	0-48	› 48	↑	
18	Cholesterol(mg/dL)	120-190	190-330	↑	
19	Triglycerides (mg/dL)	76-92	205-247	↑	
20	Renal plasma flow	420	695	↑	Increased glomerular filtration rate
21	Glomerular filtration rate (mL/min)	100±18	150±30	↑	Urinary stasis →**i**ncreased risk of urinary tract infections
22	Serum creatinine (mg/dL)	0.8-1.2	1.2-1.8	↑	
23	Blood urea nitrogen (mg/dL)	8-25	≤15	↓	

I. Musculoskeletal System

In the later stages of pregnancy, it has been seen that musculoskeletal changes are common. In late pregnancy, painful leg cramps, or ''charCharleyses,'' are some of the common complaints. Changes in calcium and phosphate metabolism lead to leg cramps.[72,73] Increases in both vascular dilation and venous stasis have both been attributed as causes of leg-muscle cramps and lower extremity edema.[74] The venous drainage from the pelvic region may also relate to the pelvis and sacroiliac pain. Due to hormonal changes, increased mobility of the sacroiliac, sacrococcygeal, and pubic joints can be seen and can hence cause lower back pain and pelvic discomfort. Weight increases may also result in a larger strain on the inter vertebral disks, leading to generalized back pain. Muscle strain and pain in the lower back can be seen in pregnant women due to the increase in the size of the gravid uterus leading to lordosis. Studies reveal that close to 49% of pregnant women experience some back pain during gestation.[72,75] A transient decrease of coordination can lead to falling and possibly a chance of minor traumas, such as contusions and bruising.

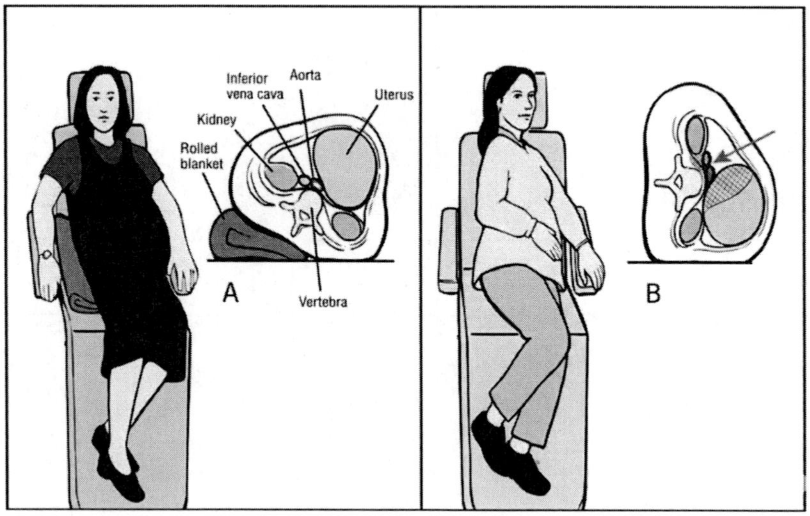

Position of pregnant patients on dental chair

II. Effects of Alcohol, Drug, or Tobacco Use

Some social habits like tobacco consumption or substance abuse are very harmful to both the patient's health and to her unborn child. Screening of all their patients should be done by medical professionals for use of tobacco, alcohol, or illegal drugs. Studies estimate that from 1.8% to 32% of pregnant women have used an illicit drug sometime during their gestation.[76-78] Medical professionals are obligated by the law of some states to report suspicion of illegal use of drugs. Thus it is important for medical professionals to know the local laws as well as their professional and ethical guidelines. The health professional should be aware of the available treatment options as well as other factors that may relate to success before suggesting to patients that they stop using tobacco, alcohol, or other drugs. In order to become successful in the same the patient motivation and desire for change are essential. For the patient's overall health and effective management, issues like underlying medical or psychological conditions are to be addressed. Additionally, consideration for treatment or counseling options, finances, and family or household obligations should be addressed.[76]

Tobacco

Premature and lower birth weights associated with tobacco use were first reported in the 1950s.[79,80] The harmful effects of tobacco on both the general population and pregnant women specifically are printed on cigarette packages since the 1970s. Tobacco cessation is of extreme importance as the known consequences of smoking include low birth weight, risks of spontaneous abortions or preterm deliveries, and increased risk of sudden infant death syndrome.[81] Animal studies have proven that both nicotine and carbon monoxide cross the placenta and cause direct effects on developing fetuses.[80,82,83] Long-term effects of tobacco have also been reported as increased risks for mental retardation and attention-deficit/hyperactivity disorder in children who were exposed to smoking in utero.[81]

While tobacco cessation is difficult for most patients, 25% to 40% of smokers report strong motivation to quit while pregnant. Of those who quit smoking, only 21% to 35% of women reported relapse during their pregnancy.[81] Successful methods for tobacco cessation include patient motivation as well as behavioral and coping counseling or the availability of educational materials.[80,84-86] For non pregnant patients, if this is not sufficient, bupropion can be used. The FDA has given bupropion a B classification for pregnancy risk.[81] Nicotine concentrates in the fetal circulation after passing the placental barrier and causes vasoconstriction of both placental and uterine blood vessels.[81,87] As such, it is an FDA category C medication and nicotine patches should only be used when their benefits clearly outweigh the risk of smoking or other cessation methods.[81]

Alcohol

It is declared by the Center for Substance Abuse Treatment that the alcohol treatment centers must prioritize pregnant women.[81,88] As only about 65% of gestational women report their alcohol consumption,[81,89] health professionals should ask all their patients about the use of alcohol. In order to find the alcoholic tendencies in a patient various standardized questionnaire have been formulated. Women who abuse alcohol while pregnant are at high risk for miscarriage or spontaneous abortion.[80] Fetal alcohol syndrome also known as FAS is a condition caused by alcohol abuse, which can lead to several physical and cognitive birth defects. Some of the facial deformities associated with FAS[80,90] are given as under:

- Cleft palate
- Visual defects
- Thin upper lips
- Absent philtrum,
- Absent epicanthal folds
- Flat midfaces

Are also reported as Some of the physical anomalies[81,91] that can be seen in FAS are given as under:

- Heart defects: ventricular septal defects
- Vertebral defects
- Hip defects,

Have been Other correlated defects associated with FAS[81] are as under:

- Lower intelligence
- Attention-deficit also known as hyperactivity disorder
- Decreased growth potential
- Failure to thrive

Cocaine and Opiate Abuse

Since the 1980s cocaine has been a common recreational drug. Cocaine is a stimulant that is associated with hypertension and peripheral vasoconstriction.[80,92] As cocaine easily crosses the placental barrier, this drug can have multiple effects on the mother as well as on the fetus. It is known to cause uterine arteries to constrict and to inhibit the metabolism of epinephrine and nor epinephrine at neural junctions.[76,80,93-95] Cocaine also increases the contractility of the pregnant woman's uterus, which may lead to uterine rupture.[76,96] In addition to this cocaine-related hypertension can also be associated with preeclampsia-like syndrome. Congenital anomalies include heart and vision defects, hydrocephaly, cerebral infarcts, and other neurological defects.[81] Children within utero cocaine exposure have been found to have attention deficit disorders during childhood and unknown effects on their maturation.[76,97] It is also a topic of concern if the fetus is under long-term narcotic exposure. Maternal narcotic dependency has been associated with low birth weights and increased neonatal mortality rates.[80] In addition to this fetal dependency on narcotics can be associated with long-term maternal usage. Neonatal symptoms may also include irritability, gastrointestinal problems, tremors, and even seizures.[76] Marijuana is another frequently abused drug, though few long-term effects have been noted for the fetus, newborn, or children.[80]

III. Infection

Pregnant women may be more susceptible than other women to infection.[97] This vulnerability can be traced in part to the physiological effects that can precipitate infections, as well as the alterations in pharmacokinetics. The increased total blood volume and vasodilation increase the dissemination of bacteria throughout the body. Also, pregnancy may alter the cell-mediated immune function, resulting in a delayed immune response to infection. Diminished gastrointestinal motility can delay peak concentration of oral medications and the increased blood volume, when combined with increased cardiac output and glomerular filtration rate, can cause rapid diffusion, but also rapid metabolism and excretion of water-soluble medications. For example, ampicillin suffers this fate, so patients receiving lower dosages may not obtain therapeutic levels of the drug.[74]

Pregnancy and Oral Health

Oral

Like any other system, the oral cavity exhibits a number of changes during pregnancy and thus requires special attention by dental care professionals.

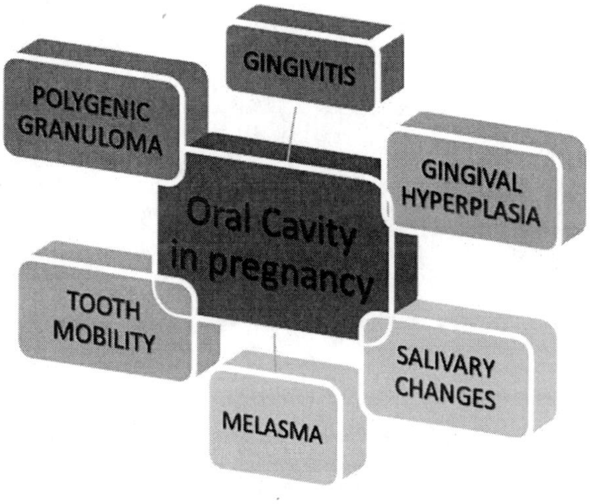

Perimylolysis (Erosion/ Decalcification of Tooth Enamel)

During pregnancy, the oral cavity gets exposed to the gastric acids that lead to erosions in the teeth. The following can be the possible reasons for the same:

Morning sickness in the first trimester can be a common cause

Acidic reflux can get increased due to a lax esophageal sphincter and the upward pressure from the gravid uterus in the later stages of pregnancy. Severe forms of erosions on the enamel can be seen in patients with severe vomiting

In order to neutralize acid[67] after vomiting following things can be done:

a) Rinsing the mouth with a fluoride mouthwash

b) Mixing baking soda with water

c) To apply casein phosphopeptide amorphous calcium phosphate also known as tooth mousse.

It is recommended that an expectant mother should not brush her teeth immediately after vomiting. They should also be instructed to use a soft or super soft (pediatric) toothbrushes in order to avoid further damage to the gastric acid exposed enamel.

Dental Caries

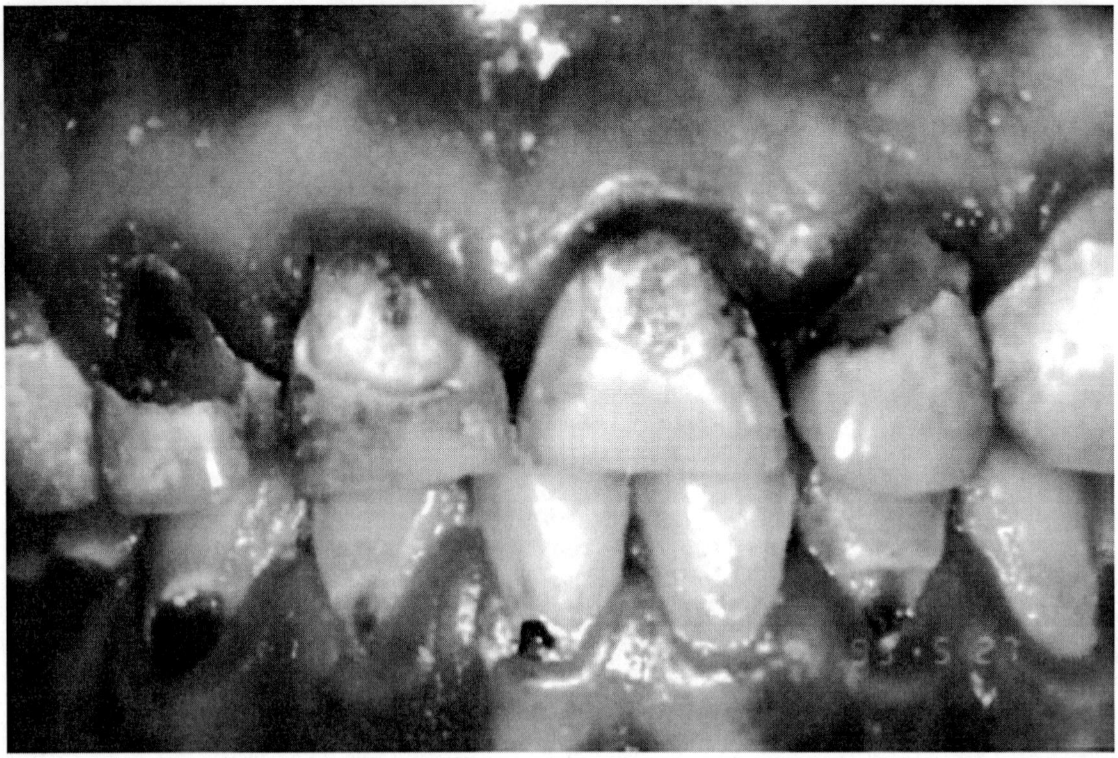

It has been documented that there is an increase in the occurrence of dental alterations has been documented, particularly caries (99.38%).[98]

Pregnant women are at a higher risk of getting caries due to the following reasons:

1) Due to frequent vomiting there is an increase in the pH in the oral cavity.
2) Cravings to have a sugary snack can be frequently seen in the expectant.
3) Oral health is neglected and gets less attention.

Local, as well as systemic complications, can be seen if an active dental caries is left untreated.

In case the infecting person which in this case is the mother has a high salivary mutans streptococci count the transmission can occur through several daily saliva contacts between the child and the mother. The attainment of mutans streptococci is said to occur during a distinct age interval called as a "window of infectivity" which is between 19 and 31 months. The proportion of children with MS increases from 25% to 75%.[99]

Pyogenic Granuloma (pregnancy tumor, or pregnancy granuloma epulis gravidarum)

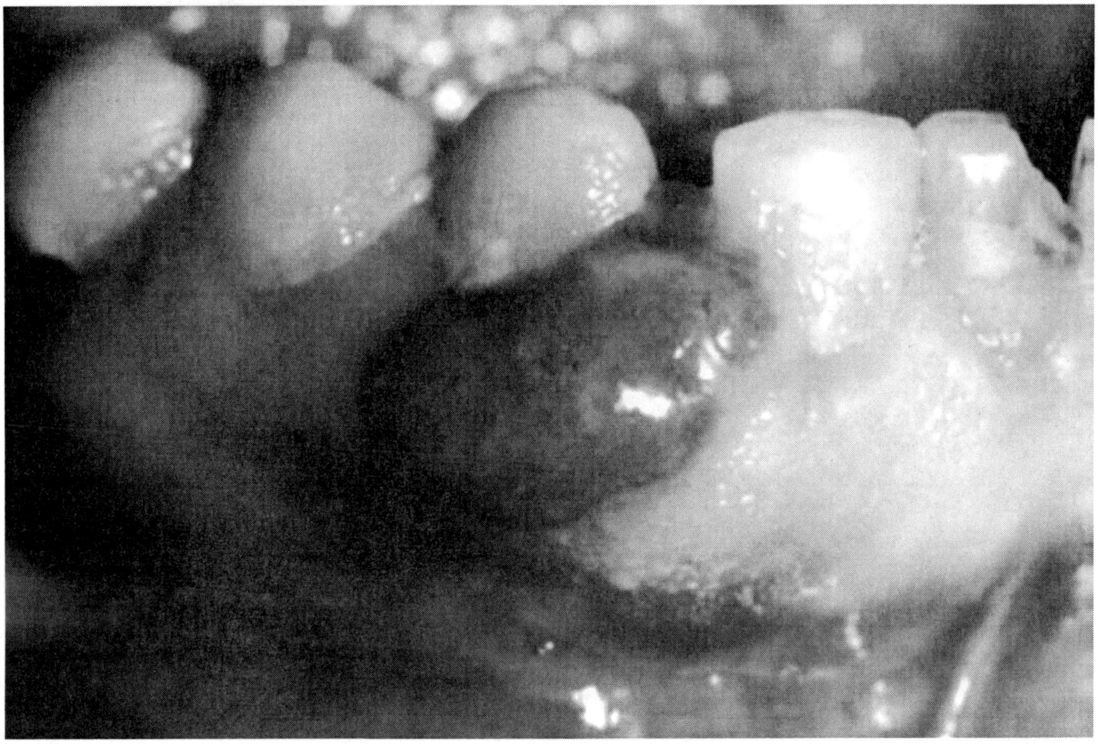

Pyogenic granuloma can be experienced by about 5% of pregnant women. Following are the factors[9,20] that are thought to cause pyogenic granuloma:

- There is an increase in localized angiogenesis due to an increase in circulating estrogen and progesterone.
- Many local factors including plaque can lead to gingival irritation.

Pyogenic granuloma can occur any time throughout the pregnancy[20] but is more common in the first or second trimester of a woman's first pregnancy.

Clinically the surface appears to be a smooth, lobulated mass that is erythematous. Gingiva is the site of its common occurrence. However, it can be found in other locations like: the tongue, palate, and the buccal mucosa. This tumor grows rapidly and usually starts to recede soon after delivery. Unless the tumor presents itself with bleeding, frequent monitoring is the first line of management. It has a higher recurrence rate if the tumor is surgically removed during the pregnancy.[100]

Gingival Hyperplasia and Pregnancy Gingivitis

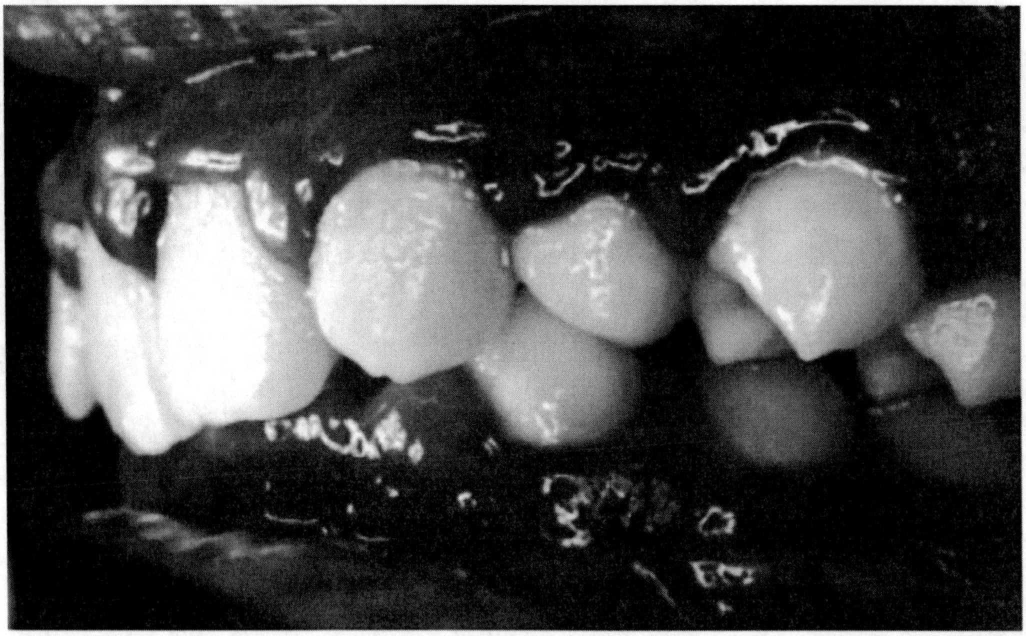

50% to 100% ofpregnancies[20,22] are accompanied by pregnancy gingivitis and/or gingival hyperplasia. Despite the absence of periodontal disease, generalized tooth mobility may also occur. The resolution is usually spontaneous after the pregnancy. Pregnancy gingivitis has the following characteristic feature:

- Dark red, swollen, smooth gingiva that bleeds easily.[22]

It starts usually in the 2nd month of the pregnancy and peaks typically in the 8th month of the pregnancy.[20]

Following changes predispose the expectant mother to pregnancy gingivitis and gingival hyperplasia:

a) As the hormones changes, the oral inflammatory process also changes.

b) Capillary permeability also increases due to an increase in the circulating estrogen.

Marginal gingiva and interdental papillae are often affected.[8] Periodontal disease is not caused by pregnancy, but it may be worsened by pregnancy.

Following are the frequent oral hygiene measures that an individual should practice in order to minimize the severity of gingivitis:

- Regular tooth brushing
- Flossing
- Use of mouthwashes

Following are the professional measures to take to minimize the severity of the gingivitis:

- Oral prophylaxis.
- Oral irrigation can minimize the severity of gingivitis.

Periodontitis

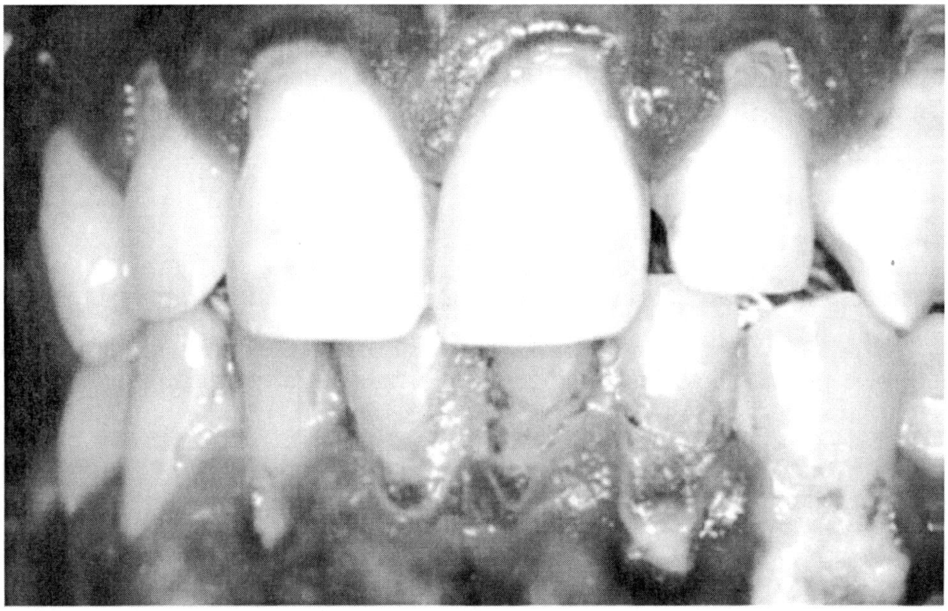

Approximately 30 percent of women of childbearing age[101] suffer from periodontitis, which is a destructive inflammation of periodontium. In this condition, the bacteria infiltrate periodontium. These bacteria produce the toxins that stimulate the chronic inflammatory response which results in the breakdown and then the destruction of periodontium creating pockets that become infected resulting in the loosening[102] of the teeth. This process can induce recurrent bacteremia, which indirectly triggers the hepatic acute phase response, resulting in the production of cytokines, prostaglandins (i.e., PGE2), and interleukins (i.e., IL-6, IL-8), all of which can affect pregnancy. In comparison to a healthy patient, the women with periodontitis show elevated levels of these inflammatory markers in the amniotic fluid of women with periodontitis and preterm birth. In one study, researchers found minimal oral bacteria in the amniotic fluid and placenta of women with preterm labor and periodontitis.[103] There is a probability that this inflammatory cascade alone prematurely initiates the labor. The release of PGE2 restricts placental blood flow and causes placental necrosis and resultant intrauterine growth restriction,[104] this mechanism is thought to be similar for low birth weight.

Periodontitis and Poor Pregnancy Outcomes

Several poor pregnancy outcomes have been seen due to periodontitis, although the mechanism by which this occurs remains unclear and is quite controversial.

Following things can be done for the management of periodontitis in pregnancy:

- Early diagnosis.
- Deep root scaling.

The American Academy of Periodontology has recommended all the women who are pregnant or who are planning to become pregnant should undergo a periodontal examination and any necessary treatment.[105]

Salivary Changes

There is a possibility that the salivary flow can be reduced during pregnancy. One study reported that 44% of pregnant women may experience persistent xerostomia. This is thought to be caused by hormonal changes.[106] Changes in salivary composition include:[8]

- Decreased sodium
- Decreased pH and increased risk of tooth demineralization
- Increased potassium
- Increased protein
- Increased salivary estrogen

Increased salivary estrogen levels may cause an increased proliferation and desquamation of the oral mucosa, along with an increased amount of gingival crevicular fluid· Desquamated oral mucosa can act as a source of nutrition for the bacteria In order to find approximate levels of plasma hormones, salivary hormone levels can be used to predict preterm birth.[8] It has been seen that the women with preterm birth have higher salivary estrogen than those who have on term delivery whereas the salivary progesterone has been found to be lower in women with preterm births as compared with women who carry to term.[107,108]

In order to treat a patient with a dry mouth, a palliative approach should be considered.To increase salivation, the patient can drink more water or chew sugarless gum or gum containing xylitol. Educate the patient on the importance of oral hygiene.[106]

Fetal Development Risks

Throughout the different stages of fetal development, different parts of the fetus go through different amounts of risk for developmental defects. There is no time when the fetus is completely safe from developing defects.

Birth Defects

Minor birth defects are present in 14% to 40% of live births.[109]

Fetal anomalies can be separated into the following three categories:[110]

1. **Malformations:** Structures that form incorrectly.
2. **Disruptions:** Destructive processes that alter structures that are already formed.
3. **Deformations:** Mechanical forces that mold or shape portions of the fetus over time.

Principles of Teratology

A teratogen is something that has been found to cause birth defects. The factors that contribute to the ability of something to produce birth defects are also known as the principles of teratology. The susceptibility of the teratogen depends partly on the fetal genotype and also on the maternal genome. Maternal metabolism of drugs and immune system function (resistance to infection) both play a role in the susceptibility of the fetus to a teratogen.[110]

The stage of fetal development when the exposure occurs affects the impact of the exposure on the fetus.[109] Embryogenesis is from the 3rd to the 8th week of fetal development after fertilization. This is when the fetus is most susceptible to birth defects. Each organ system may have multiple periods or moments when exposure to a teratogen may lead to a defect in that organ system. The severity of the birth defect can depend on both the dose and the duration of exposure to a teratogen. Teratogens have specific mechanisms by which they induce birth defects.

Teratogens can cause abnormal development that may result in[109] the following:

- Growth retardation
- Death
- Malformation
- Functional disorders

A drug is classified as a teratogen if it has the potential to produce a developmental abnormality. A common example is thalidomide. If 50 mg of thalidomide is given on the 26th day of pregnancy, there is a significant risk to the embryo. However, thalidomide does not always harm the fetus. If the same 50 mg of thalidomide is given during the 10th week of pregnancy, structural malformations are not expected. Similarly, 1 mg of thalidomide given any time during pregnancy is not expected to have an effect on the fetus or embryo.[110]

The Timing of Teratogen Exposure

The most critical period for brain development is 3 to 16 weeks post-conception. (However, the brain may still be affected by teratogens after this period.)[110] During weeks 5 and 6 Cleft lip development is most sensitive. Enamel development is most sensitive during the end of week 6 through week 8: Enamel hypoplasia and staining can occur because of problems during this time frame. Tooth development is sensitive from week 9 onward. Cleft palate development is most sensitive during the end of week 6 through the beginning of week 9.62.

Types of Teratogens

Dentistry potentially overlaps with a number of these categories of teratogens. Because dentistry addresses certain maternal diseases, providing dental care may reduce teratogen exposure. On the other hand, there may be a concern that dental care may be unsafe because it includes potentially teratogenic components (eg, x-rays, medications, and dental materials).

Teratogens can be placed into a number of different categories, as follows:

- Infectious agents that include rubella, herpes simplex, cytomegalovirus, varicella
- Physical agents that include, x-rays, hyperthermia
- Chemical agents that includes thalidomide, phenytoin, lithium, alcohol
- Hormones
- Maternal disease
- Nutritional deficiencies
- Hypoxia
- Heavy metals (eg, organic mercury and lead)

Fetal Development

The first 2 weeks after fertilization, or 2 to 4 weeks after the last menstruation is termed as Predifferentiation. Resistance to teratogenic effects is seen during this period. However, there may be problems with zygote cleavage or blastocyst implantation or early spontaneous abortion of the embryo.[109]

The Embryonic Period (Embryogenesis)

The embryonic period is from 5 to 10 weeks after last menstruation or 3 to 8 weeks after fertilization.[110] After 2-8 weeks after fertilization major organogenesis. During this period, major malformations can occur.[110] This is the time period when the embryo is most at risk for teratogenesis.[20,22]

The Fetal Period (Fetogenesis)

The fetal period goes from week 11 after last menstruation to birth (or week 9 after fertilization to birth.)[110] Few structural defects or malformations occur during this period.

This period however can show deformations and disruptions. Throughout pregnancy central nervous system development remains vulnerable to teratogens.

Fetal Loss

Between 50% and 75% of all spontaneous abortions occur during the first trimester or the time from conception up to the 14th week of gestation.[8] A fetus with a major chromosomal abnormality usually does not last until the 14th week of pregnancy. During weeks 14 through 23 of pregnancy, the risk of pregnancy loss is 1% to 2%. Causes for fetal loss during the second trimester include inflammation of fetal membranes, inflammation of the umbilical cord, and viral infection of the placenta.[106]

Pregnancy and Oral Health Screening

Screening for pregnancy

A. All women of child bearing age should be asked the following screening questions to assess the possibility of pregnancy.[20,111]

- Are you pregnant?
- Is there any possibility that you are pregnant and are unaware of it?
- Are you trying to get pregnant?

B. Assessing reproductive history

The number of times a woman has become pregnant regardless of the outcome[112]is known as gravidity or gravida. is The number that refers to pregnancy outcomes is known as parity or para.The meaning of parity may differ.

GTPAL

The GTPAL that stands for gravida, term, premature, abortions, living children is a system that contains five numbers that summarize a woman's reproductive history:

- **G:** Regardless of the outcome, how many times a woman has become pregnant
- **T:** Term births (number)
- **P:** Premature births (number)

- **A:** Total number of abortions, miscarriages, or ectopic pregnancies
- **L:** Number of living children

Assessing oral health

For the oral health assessment, ask questions similar to the following:[22,113]

- When and where did you last visit a dentist?
- Are your gums swollen? Do they bleed?
- Do you have any toothache or pain?
- Do you experience any problems while eating or chewing food?
- Do you experience any other problems in your mouth?
- Do you have any symptoms that indicate a high-risk pregnancy eg, high blood pressure,prior miscarriages, recent cramping, or bleeding?
- How many weeks pregnant are you? What trimester are you in? When is your due date?
- Do you have any concerns or queries about getting oral health care during your pregnancy?
- During the course of your pregnancy, have you been vomiting? If so, how frequently?
- Have you getting care for your pregnancy?

Guideline for dental treatment

Following are the four categories of dental treatment:

a) Emergency.

b) Urgent.

c) Necessary.

d) Elective.[112,114]

Emergency Dental Treatment

The treatment for a condition that requires immediate attention for the patient's oral and/or systemic well-being is known as emergency dental treatment. We will consider a condition a dental emergency if it is either an acute injury or illness in which there is an immediate risk to a patient's life or long-term dental health.

Following are some conditions that require immediate dental treatment:

- **Oral Hemorrhage:** The patient, in this case, may bleed to death, and hence it must be controlled in time.
- **Ludwig Angina:** this condition may compromise the patient's ability to breathe hence can be a potentially life-threatening infection that targets the floor of the mouth.
- **Traumatic Injury:** The patient can receive treatment in an emergency or urgent care center, depending on the severity of the accident. If the patient has a minor injury eg, an avulsed tooth they can go to a dental office. In the case of an avulsed tooth, there is a limited amount of time in which the tooth may be able to be re-implanted.

Urgent Dental Treatment

Urgent dental treatment would be considered a treatment for conditions where the patient is experiencing significant symptoms. A small delay in treatment is not expected to significantly affect the treatment outcome.

Conditionincludes:

- Symptomatic irreversible pulpitis
- Cracked tooth syndrome
- Dental abscess,
- It should also be noted that severe abscesses and infections may require emergency treatment.

Necessary Dental Treatment

A treatment that can improve the health of the pregnant woman or fetus during the time course of pregnancy is called necessary dental treatment.

Condition includes:

- Fractured tooth causing minor pain.
- If the pregnant woman undergoes general anesthesia at the time of the delivery, periodontally compromised teeth can be avulsed and aspirated during intubation.
- During the time of pregnancy, caries that is either symptomatic or suspected to become symptomatic.
- Asymptomatic irreversible pulpitis.

Elective Dental Treatment

During the time of pregnancy if the treatment does not affect the health of the pregnant woman or the fetus it is said to be elective dental care. Oral pathologies are not necessarily treated in elective dental treatment. An example of this is: cosmetic surgeries Such type of treatment should be deferred till the end of the pregnancy.

Conditions include:

- Oral pathologies that are difficult to treat during pregnancy and can spontaneously resolve after pregnancy

A good example for this is: If an asymptomatic pyogenic granuloma of pregnancy is removed during pregnancy[112,114] it may reoccur.

- Cosmetic surgery
- Veneers (no caries)
- Tooth whitening
- Small cracks in composites and amalgam having no caries
- Tiny caries lesions

When to Provide Dental Care

Ideally, all necessary dental treatment should have been completed before the pregnancy. Generally, the safest option is to defer all the dental treatment after the pregnancy, when there is no fetal risk. However, if it is an emergency it is recommended to provide urgent dental treatment even during the pregnancy. Some of the conditions in which a pregnant patient should get treatment even during the pregnancy are acute infections and abscesses.[115,116,22,112,113,117-121] Both the type of treatment and the phase of pregnancy should be taken into consideration while providing treatment.

While giving a dental treatment[114] it should be taken into account that deferring elective, nonessential, and postponable treatment until after pregnancy eliminates the possibility any fetal risk. Pregnancy is finite and relatively short, lasting only 9 to 10 months in length, and most oral pathologies are slowly progressing, non–life-threatening, and benign.[115,114] Dental care can often be postponed until either the second trimester or after delivery.[115,111,122]

Safety Considerations

Pregnancy itself is not a contraindication to dental care.[123] "Evidence has failed to show any improvement in outcomes after dental treatment during pregnancy. Nonetheless, these studies did not raise any concern about the safety of dental services during pregnancy."According to the American College of Obstetricians and Gynecologists,[124] A healthy pregnant woman having a normal pregnancy should have her urgent and emergency dental needs taken care of at any time during pregnancy.[115,124,116,113,117-121] The decision of dental treatment in a hospital or an outpatient dental office setting will depend on the patient's health and the type and extent of the oral pathology.[121]

Consequences of Dental Treatment

The full impact of treatment is potentially not known, when it comes to developing fetus for many years. Severe complications of dental treatment can occur, though they are rare. At the extreme, death has occurred in the dental office Some examples of severe iatrogenic-related complications include adverse reactions or allergies to medication as well as aspiration. Aspiration of dental instruments or dental materials is a life-threatening event and can cause significant medical complications. Treatment may require a hospital-based multidisciplinary team.[124] Things as common as full-arch dental impressions may place the patient at risk for aspirating the impression material and swallowed object shave the risk of causing perforation of the gastrointestinal tract. An additional treatment may be required in case the treatment does not go as planned. Fetus may be at increased risk due to this additional treatment. In addition, there are psychological risks that may affect both the patient and the dentist. For example, the expectant mother may reach the conclusion that dental treatment was the cause of an adverse pregnancy outcome. While uncommon, a woman may take legal action against the provider in the absence of scientific evidence supporting her belief.[22]

Determining Needs for Treatment

Severe odontogenic infection imposes a small risk of death to the pregnant woman, and hence to the fetus. These cases require urgent referral and treatment in a hospital capable of multidisciplinary treatment, including surgical, anesthetic, and obstetric services.[121] On the other hand, delaying elective treatment may prevent dental treatment from being correlated with fetal demise.[20]

Aspiration

In order to decrease the risk of aspiration that may occur if a pregnant woman needs to be placed under general anesthesia either at delivery or for some other reason during her pregnancy is one of the reason why we should provide dental treatment. Poor oral health may lead to conditions that cause aspiration during intubation.[113]

Some examples include:

- Tooth fragments that can be from fractured teeth or severely decayed teeth
- Periodontally compromised teeth that become dislodged
- Temporary crowns

- Other dental materials

Timing of Treatment

In general, oral pathologies that may cause pain or infection during the time course of pregnancy should be treated during pregnancy.[124] When possible, place definitive restoration during pregnancy to minimize aspiration risk should intubation become necessary.[113]

Some reasons to consider deferring dental treatment include the following:

- The patient has a medical condition that places her or the fetus at risk if she under goes dental treatment.
- The patient has a history or elevated risk of miscarriage.
- During pregnancy certain pathologies may recur when treated and resolve after pregnancy. An example is a pregnancy-related pyogenic granuloma.[112,114]

Comprehensive dental treatment plan

Create a comprehensive dental treatment plan for the patient that includes:[22,113]

- Chief complaint
- Health history
- History of substance use (including tobacco and alcohol)
- Clinical evaluation
- Caries risk assessment
- Periodontal disease risk assessment
- Comprehensive periodontal examination (with periodontal charting)
- Any maintenance therapy that may be required during the course pregnancy

Definitive diagnoses required for dental treatment can be obtained by performing diagnostic tests

Medical Consults

To minimize risk, it is important to assess the health of the woman and her pregnancy.[116] A physician consult is not required when providing routine dental treatment to a healthy pregnant woman, but it may serve as a tool that can help educate the patient that it is safe to get dental care during the period of pregnancy.

Consider a consultation with the patient's prenatal care provider in the following situations:[124,22,113,117,120]

- **When making the decision:** whether or not to defer necessary dental treatment till after the pregnancy.
- When treatment may require the use of nitrous oxide, intravenous sedation, or general anesthesia.
- When co-morbid medical conditions such as pulmonary problems, heart or valvular disease,, bleeding disorders, diabetes,, and heparin-treated thrombophilia and hypertension.

Dental Treatment-Inducedbacteremia

Transient bacteremia often follows dental treatment.[20,22] While the effects of this bacteremia have not been well studied, clinical trials have not reported adverse effects from bacteremia that was induced by dental treatment.

Procedure Guidelines

First Trimester Recommendations: Conception through week 13

The first trimester is considered the most critical time period of gestation because organogenesis is occurring during this time.[20,22,136] The majority of spontaneous abortions (85%) occur during the first trimester.[125] Hence, dental treatment should be limited to emergency and urgent treatments. When possible, provide definitive treatment.[112,118,119] Routine radiograph should be avoided and selective radiographs should be performed as needed to diagnose oral diseases that require immediate treatment.[8,20,105,113] Periodontal prophylaxis can be done, but the second trimester is the preferred time to provide a dental prophylaxis.[8,113]

Provide patient education and anticipatory guidance that includes educating the patient about oral changes during pregnancy and also what to expect after pregnancy. Provide oral hygiene instructions for plaque control.[22,112]

Second-Trimester Recommendations: Week 14 through week 26

The second trimester, specifically weeks 14 to 20, is the preferred time to provide dental treatment during pregnancy.[8,115,124,116,20,22,112-114,117-120] There is less risk of pregnancy loss during this time frame when compared with the first trimester, and organogenesis is complete. Because the fetus is smaller than it will be at term and the uterus is below the umbilicus until about week 20, the woman will likely be more comfortable compared with later in pregnancy.

Provide dental treatment to control active oral diseases and urgent pathologies.[115,116,22,112,113,117-119] Provide scaling, polishing, and curettage as clinically indicated.[8] Avoid routine radiographs, but take select radiographs when needed.[8,20,118]

From the middle of the second trimester on, position the patient on her left side during treatment to minimize the risk of supine hypotension.[116,22,120]

Provide patient education, including oral hygiene instructions and anticipatory guidance to inform the patient about oral changes during pregnancy and also what to expect after pregnancy.[22,112]

In the sixth month of pregnancy, it has been suggested that the expectant mother should start using a daily mouth rinse of 0.05% sodium fluoride and 0.12% chlorhexidine. The purpose is to improve maternal oral health through the reduction of caries-causing bacteria. This in turn may delay colonization of caries-causing bacteria in the infant after delivery.[106]

Third Trimester Recommendations: Week 27 until delivery

By the third trimester, the end of pregnancy is nearing. In general, the safest option is to defer dental treatment until after pregnancy. It is better to provide dental care in the first half of the third trimester if the treatment is necessary. Dental care should be deferred from the middle of the third trimester until a few weeks postpartum.[8,106]

Provide oral hygiene instructions and anticipatory guidance on what to expect after pregnancy.[22,112] If dental treatment is performed, provide dental care that is needed to improve the health of the expectant mother and baby during pregnancy.[115,124,116,22,112,113,121] When needed, take select radiographs.[8,118,120] Consider short dental appointments to minimize patient discomfort that may be present because of her enlarged uterus. Also, patients should be positioned on their left side to minimize the risk of supine hypotension.[116,22,112]

Immediate postpartum recommendations: Dental care is usually best deferred until a few weeks after birth. Unless the woman has had significant blood loss during delivery, she is in a hypercoagulable state for at least 2 to 3 weeks after delivery.[116] Epinephrine may increase the risk of coagulation.

Dental Radiographs

Radiographs should only be taken when it is thought that the diagnostic yield will affect patient care.[106,126] Dental radiographs expose patients to an extremely small amount of radiation.This small amount minimizes the risk of harm to the patient and the fetus, but the risk cannot be completely eliminated. However, the diagnostic information from clinically indicated, properly taken dental radiographs is generally considered to outweigh the risk of harm.[106] Digital radiographs expose the patient to a fraction of the radiation required for traditional film radiographs.[20,22]

Effect of radiation on the fetus

Following are the two factors affects the effect of radiation on fetus:

- The gestation of the fetus and
- The dose of radiation.

Fetal cells are actively dividing during the first trimester as a result of which is most sensitive to radiation during this period. During the second and third trimesters,the fetus is less sensitive to radiation.[8,113,127]

If the estimated threshold dosage of teratogenicity is correct, the risk of teratogenesis from dental x-ray exposure should be virtually nonexistent (< 0.1%). The risk of spontaneous abortion or malformation is 1,000 times greater.[20]

The American College of Radiology and the American College of Obstetricians and Gynecologists have both made the statement that the radiation dose for a single diagnostic procedure is insufficient to cause harm to a developing embryo or fetus.[120] With properly functioning modern equipment, it is unlikely that the abdominal area will be exposed to x-rays when taking dental radiographs. Because of this, the benefit of shielding the abdominal area with a lead apron is likely to be primarily psychological. However, the ADA currently recommends the use of a lead apron to shield both the thyroid and the abdominal areas.[8]

Effect On Dental Treatment

The benefit of taking necessary dental radiographs to diagnose and treat a disease that requires immediate treatment is thought to outweigh the risk, particularly for otherwise healthy expectant mothers.[106]

The American Dental Association (ADA) and Food and Drug Administration (FDA) guidelines state that before conducting a radiographic examination, a dentist should do the following:[126]

- Conduct a clinical examination.
- Oral and medical histories should be considered for patients with medical histories.
- Consider the patient's vulnerability to environmental factors that may affect her oral health.
- Prescribe an individualized radiographic examination.

Both the ADA and the National Council on Radiation Protection and Measurements recommend that if treatment will be done after delivery, dental radiographs should also be taken after delivery.[106]

Reasons to Take Radiographs During Pregnancy

Both incomplete and inaccurate diagnoses can lead to inadequate or inappropriate treatment, appropriate dental radiographs should be taken during pregnancy.[8] Radiographs should be taken when the standard of care includes radiographs and when treatment cannot wait until after delivery.[20,119] However, radiographs should only be taken when there is an expectation that the diagnostic yield will affect patient care.[106,126]

The dentist has the responsibility to adhere to the ALARA (as low as reasonably achievable) principle and minimize the radiation exposure of the patient.[120,126]

Some ways to minimize radiation exposure include:[8]

- Avoid radiographs during pregnancy, especially during the first trimester, unless there is a clinical reason.[119]
- Take bitewing instead of panoramic radiographs.
- Use high-speed film or digital x-rays. Image receptors or film speeds slower than the American National Standards Institute speed group E should be avoided.
- Use rectangular collimation instead of circular collimation.
- Use a properly collimated beam.
- Use a lead apron that covers the abdomen and has a protective thyroid collar on the neck.[119]

Dental Materials

Dentists are fortunate to have a profession where they are able to quickly improve the quality of people's lives every day. However, this comes with the responsibility to have an awareness of the impacts of restoring teeth using various dental materials.At this time, little is known about the safety of using dental fillings during pregnancy. Research has found that both amalgam and composite fillings can affect the human body, but this research has been insufficient to determine how this may affect fetal development. In general, it is thought that the benefit outweighs the risk when treating symptomatic oral conditions or conditions that may become symptomatic during pregnancy.[124]

Fetal Exposure to Dental Materials

The use of a rubber dam for isolation during restorative procedures helps to minimize maternal ingestion, aspiration, and inhalation of dental materials.[124,22,113,123] Although little is known about the safety of using dental materials during pregnancy, the FDA classifies dental fillings (including encapsulated amalgam, gold, and composite fillings)as a class II medical device (moderate risk.[22,113]) If the FDA pregnancy rating for drugs were applied to dental fillings; they would likely be classified as Category B Dental amalgam.

Fetal Exposure to Mercury Through a Dental Amalgam

Organic mercury (found in the environment) and inorganic mercury (found in dental materials) are two general forms of mercury that are both well-known neurotoxins.[22,128] Exposure to inorganic mercury from dental materials typically occurs at a much lower rate than exposure to organic mercury from the environment.[46] Dental amalgam contains about 50% inorganic mercury.[120,129] A person with amalgam restorations is exposed to mercury vapor (Hg0) throughout the life of the restorations, but the threshold level in which Hg0 exposure causes neurotoxicity is not known.[129] The World Health Organization (WHO) estimates the maximum total safe mercury intake to be 2 µg/kg/d, and the amount of mercury released from dental amalgams in the mouth is estimated to be approximately 10 µg/d. Factoring in body weight, this is well under the WHO's estimated maximum.

Germany, Austria, and Canada have chosen to restrict the placing of amalgam restorations in pregnant women. Other countries, including Sweden and Denmark, are choosing to phase out amalgam altogether due to environmental Concerns.[113]

Fetal Accumulation Of Mercury

Mercury oxide (Hg0) may be inhaled and absorbed into the bloodstream and crosses the placental Barrier.[120] Mercury concentration in umbilical cord blood is similar to that of the expectant mother, and higher concentrations have been found in fetal kidneys compared with fetal brains.[128] Fetal brain accumulation of Hg appears to be less than that found in the pregnant woman's brain.[129] This appears to be because the fetal liver converts Hg0into Hg++, which does not cross the blood-brain barrier as easily as Hg0.

Mercury vapor

Hg0 may be released and systemically absorbed during the following events:[22]

- When placing and removing amalgam restorations.
- Bruxing and chewing on amalgam restorations.
- When whitening teeth with products that use or generate hydrogen peroxide in the presence of amalgam restorations.[106]

Aside from rare hypersensitivity reactions, the following organizations have made statements that current evidence does not support the concern that dental amalgams are unsafe.[130]

- American Dental Association

- Alzheimer's Association
- American Academy of Pediatrics
- Autism Society of America
- US Environmental Protection Agency
- Mayo Clinic
- National Multiple Sclerosis Society
- Food and Drug Administration
- New England Journal of Medicine
- International Journal of Dentistry
- National Council Against Health Fraud
- National Institute of Dental and Cranio-facial Research
- American Cancer Society
- Web MD

There is no correlation found between the number of amalgam fillings in the mother and the mercury concentration in human breast milk.

Effect On Dental Treatment

Studies have not found adverse reproductive effects resulting from the placement,removal, or presence of dental amalgam[120]. In the absence of pathology, deferring the elective replacement of dental amalgam restorations with composite restorations may further minimize fetal exposure to mercury. Consider deferring the use of tooth whitening products that use or generate hydrogen peroxide until after pregnancy because they may cause inorganic mercury to be released from dental amalgams.[22,106]

Composite Resin

Composite resins are made up of polymerized resin (methacrylate monomers) and inorganic fillers. Research on methacrylate monomers shows that after polymerization, some monomers may be released into the oral cavity and also diffuse through the dentin to the dental pulp.[22] Bisphenol A (BPA) is a chemical that can be used to make hard plastics and dental composite resins. High concentrations of BPA have been shown to cause health problems, and there is a concern that BPA may be present when using dental sealants and composite restorations.[131,132]

Effect on Dental Treatment

There are no known short-term health risks with the placement of dental sealants or composite resins. However, there is also insufficient information available to determine if there are any effects of long-term exposure.[22] Dental composite resins have not been shown to adversely affect health through exposure to BPA.[131]

Scaling and Root Planning (SRP) and Prophylaxis During Pregnancy

Periodontal disease is correlated with a variety of adverse pregnancy outcomes. These adverse outcomes may include low birth weight (LBW), preterm birth (PTB), small size for gestational age, pregnancy-induced hypertension, and fetal loss. The cause-effect relationships between pregnancy and periodontal disease have not yet been established; periodontal disease may lead to pregnancy complications, pregnancy may worsen the periodontal disease, or the two may build off each other.[66]

Ideally, a woman should be free of periodontal disease prior to becoming pregnant. Nonsurgical periodontal therapy such as SRP may benefit the patient. There is conflicting evidence as to whether the fetus will benefit if the patient under goes periodontal treatment. There may be certain categories of high-risk pregnancies where there is a possible fetal benefit to receiving periodontal therapy during pregnancy. Further research is needed to confirm and identify which women may benefit from receiving periodontal treatment during pregnancy.[66] The fetal benefit may be linked to the success of periodontal therapy. The timing of periodontal therapy during the pregnancy may affect whether or not there is a fetal benefit.

Effect on Dental Treatment

Researchers suggest that it is safe to provide SRP and dental prophylaxis during pregnancy.[66] The safest time for SRP is considered to be the The first half of the second trimester. One research study found no increased risk of adverse medical events when SRP is done during this time frame. Additional factors such as the may need to be taken into consideration When recommending treatment options, additional factors such as woman's health and her ability to tolerate treatment should also be taken into consideration.

Antibiotic prophylaxis is not routinely recommended to address the treatment-induced bacteremia during pregnancy. Antibiotic prophylaxis may be given for other clinically indicated reasons, such as the presence of multiple infections. When anesthetic agents are needed, consider pregnancy category B anesthetics.

Consider lidocaine or a lidocaine/ prilocaine combination (eg, Oraqix [Dentsply]) for topical anesthesia. Consider lidocaine with 1:100,000 epinephrine for local anesthesia.

Drug Administration During Pregnancy

During a woman's pregnancy medications can either be a boon or liability. This can be determined by evaluating and balancing the following:

a) Weight of her medical condition.

b) The fetus's exposure risk.

c) The need for medical treatment.

Some physicians, dental professionals, or even patients may believe that all medications may be harmful to the unborn child which tends to be an irrational fear. Whereas there are some medical conditions that if left untreated may be more detrimental to the fetus. This may lead to the following things:

- Progressive Maternal Disease Status
- Teratogenesis
- Impaired Fetal Growth Or Development
- Premature Birth
- Spontaneous Miscarriage
- Abortion

There are many safe alternatives that can be given to pregnant patients in order to treat these medical conditions which are not harmful to the fetus.An informed choice has to be made by both the patient and the medical professional. Once the decision for medical management has been made, the selection of a medication must be balanced by the following:

✓ Therapeutic options available

✓ The degree of control that is required for a medical condition

✓ The potential and degree of exposure to the fetus

✓ Risks of various medications on fetus and mother

✓ Dosages necessary for control and safety

✓ Long-term effects of the medication on the fetus

There are few controlled studies conducted due to ethical concerns suggesting the adverse effects of medications on either human fetuses or future development and maturation of the child and adult. Various circumstantial reports are present reflecting adverse effects of medication and do not adequately reflect a drug's safety status. A reliable rule of thumb may include reviewing non-pharmacologic treatments, becoming familiar with current pharmacologic standards of care, and considering older pharmaceutical treatments that have a long record of safety.

The FDA considers a number of the medications commonly used in dentistry to be relatively safe. However, a risk-benefit evaluation should be considered before prescribing or administering any medication to a pregnant patient.[133] If a woman is trying to become pregnant, she should be advised of the potential risk if she becomes pregnant while taking a medication.

When selecting a medication to administer or prescribe, the dentist should consider the following:[106,133]

- Evaluate the potential risk and benefit to expectant mother and her unborn baby.
- Choose the medication most likely to be safest.
- Minimize the duration and dosage.

Factors That Affect the Bioavailability of Drugs to the Fetus

Maternal plasma has a higher capacity to bind drugs than fetal plasma, but this difference has not been shown to be significant for toxicity.[21] Drugs that compete for plasma protein binding may be more bioavailable to fetal plasma, and fetal acidemia may lead to increased drug absorption and retention in the placenta.[31] Only free, unbound drugs are able to travel to the placenta.[22]

Several factors predispose the patient to fetal exposure to unbound drugs[8] during pregnancy:

- Decreased serum concentration required for drug binding
- Increased drug distribution volume
- Decreased maximum plasma concentration
- Decreased plasma half-life
- Increased lipid solubility
- Increased clearance of drugs
- Delayed gastric emptying (which may in turn increase drug bioavailability)[22]

The chance of accidental intravascular injection is present as the injection for nerve blocks occurs right next to blood vessels. A drug systemically as a result of Accidental intravascular injection. With proper technique, the chance of accidental intravascular injection is minimized.[21,123] With respect to the human lifetime, studies on pregnant women are been conducted over very short time frames, as a result of which it may take many years before the adverse effects become apparent. For example, if in-utero exposure to a drug caused a minor decrease in intelligence or fertility, it may not be noticed for many years, if at all.[133]

Nursing Mothers

A single prescription may overlap pregnancy, birth, and nursing. It is important to be aware that the nursing infant is exposed to most maternal drugs via breast milk.[20,8] Because of this, it is best to educate a woman taking prescription medicine while nursing about the possible risks of the said medicine.

FDA Pregnancy Risk Categories

FDA pregnancy risk categories (PRCs) are a useful tool that is used to determine what medications to provide to pregnant patients.The FDA has replaced PRCs with the Pregnancy and Lactation Labeling Rule (PLLR) for prescription drugs[87] as PRCs are over simplified and may lead to poorly informed clinical decisions.

FDA pregnancy categories[99]

- Adequate,well-controlled studies in pregnant women have failed to demonstrate a risk to the fetus in the first trimester of pregnancy, and there is no evidence of a risk in later trimesters. There is a remote possibility that this drug can harm the fetus. Because studies cannot rule out the possibility of harm, however, this drug should be used during pregnancy only if clearly needed.
- Despite the fact that there are no adequate and well-controlled studies in pregnant women however the animal reproduction studies have failed to demonstrate a risk to the fetus. Animal reproduction studies have shown an adverse effect (other than decreased infertility), but adequate and well-controlled studies done on pregnant women over the course of time has failed to demonstrate a risk to the fetus during the first trimester and there has been no evidence that supports the of risk in later trimesters as the animal reproduction studies are not always predictive of human response and because the studies in humans cannot rule out the possibility of harm, this drug should be used in pregnancy only if clearly needed.
- There are no adequate and well-controlled studies in humans, and either there are no animal reproduction studies that have shown an adverse effect on the fetus.It is also not known whether this drug can cause fetal harm when administered to a pregnant woman or if it can affect reproduction capacity. Despite the potential risks of these drugs on pregnant women, the benefits from the use of the drug may be acceptable. If the potential benefits of this drug justify the potential risks to the fetus only then this drug should be used during pregnancy.
- Based on adverse reaction data from investigational or marketing experience or studies in humans has been seen that there is positive evidence of human fetal risk, but despite the potential risks, the potential benefits from the use of the drug in pregnant women may be acceptable.

Inadvertent exposure to a drug is also not addressed by this labeling. Because about 50% of pregnancies are unplanned, there is significant potential for inadvertent drug exposure. Potential developmental toxicities cannot be adequately addressed by labeling, which may include:

- Fetal death
- Structural malformations
- Perturbations of fetal growth
- Functional deficits

There should In order to include human exposure information a mechanism should routinely update the Pregnancy subsection of Labeling.

PLLR

The FDA is phasing out pregnancy categories A, B, C, D, and X.[118] The new system, PLLR, gives a risk summary of the drug being that has been used during pregnancy and lactation, it also tells how a particular drug may affect reproductive potential. It is important to be aware that the PLLR only applies to prescription medications, not over-the-counter medications.[118]

This new labeling replaces the simplified single-letter representation of risk which was provided by PRCs in the past with a more informative narrative.

The FDA has chosen to phase out the PRCs for prescription medications because the PLLR will better support the needs of clinicians to safely treat patients.[118] However, clinicians will likely still encounter the PRCs in their practice during the transition to the PLLR, and the PRCs will remain for over-the-counter medications. By identifying the limitations of the PRCs, the clinician will have a greater understanding of the implications of using them to prescribe or administer medications to the pregnant patient.

The PRC classification system may incorrectly convey that drug risk categories increase from A to X as drugs are determined to carry greater risk. Categories C, D, and X may all have similar risks but they are categorized differently based on different risk-benefit considerations. This classification system may also incorrectly lead the practitioner to conclude that the drugs from the same category have a similar risk for developmental toxicity. Currently, drugs with known risks can be placed in the same category as drugs with no known risk.

The following things are to taken into account in the PRC labeling:

- Whether the risk is based on effects that have been observed in human versus animal studies.
- Statistical significance and study design.
- Degree of risk based on dose, duration, frequency, route of exposure, or gestational timing.

Medications

Non-steroidal Anti-Inflammatory Drugs

NSAIDs inhibit prostaglandin synthesis, which may lead to the following risks:[21,8]

- Delayed labor. Prostaglandins act on the endometrial lining and help induce labor. Inhibiting prostaglandin synthesis may delay labor, prolong labor (dystocia), and prolong pregnancy.[20,8,115]
- Miscarriage.[8,40]
- The ductus arteriosus closes prematurely in the fetus.

This can cause:

a) Pulmonary hypertension,

b) Respiratory problems,

c) Renal dysfunction,

d) Hemostatic abnormalities.[20,8,21]

Cyclooxygenase-2 (COX2) inhibitors are a category of NSAIDs that act on the COX2 enzyme. The COX2 enzyme is involved in one of the major pain and inflammation pathways and is involved with the conversion of arachidonic acid into prostaglandin H2.[20]

Considerations During Pregnancy

In general, NSAIDs are not recommended during pregnancy.[20,115,134] NSAIDs that are more frequently used in pregnancy include ibuprofen, naproxen, and ketoprofen.[124]

- If NSAIDs are prescribed, some general considerations include the following:
- Use the lowest effective dose.[8]
- Minimize the duration of use and limit use to 48 to 72 hours.[22,106,124]
- Avoid use in the first trimester, third trimester, and just after delivery.[45,12,125]
- Consider the pregnancy risk category (PRC).

Some consider NSAIDs, s-+

uch as ibuprofen and naproxen, to be PRC B during the first and second trimester.[20]

- COX2 inhibitors are classified as PRC C.[20]
- NSAIDs are classified as PRC D during the third trimester.[20]

Considerations for Nursing Mothers

COX2 inhibitors have a long half-life and should be avoided in breastfeeding mothers.[44] The package insert for ibuprofen recommends to either stop nursing or stop taking the medication.[135] While some consider ibuprofen to be safe during breastfeeding, small amounts of NSAIDs are found in breast milk, thereby placing the infant at slight risk.[8,20]

Opioids

Opioids are centrally acting analgesics and should be used with caution.[20,21] Be aware of the potential for addiction and drug abuse when prescribing opioids.[20] Opioids pass from the pregnant woman to the fetus.[8] While the short duration of low-dose narcotics has not been shown to cause fetal anomalies, chronic use of opioids during pregnancy may lead to the following:[20,115]

- Premature delivery
- Growth retardation
- Physical dependency (fetal and maternal)
- Neonatal narcotic withdrawal syndrome
- Depression of the fetal central nervous system
- Depression of the fetal respiratory system

Considerations During Pregnancy

When indicated, certain opioid analgesics can be used during both pregnancy and lactation.[8]

The dentist may consider consulting with the patient's prenatal care provider prior to prescribing opioids.[20] When acetaminophen provides insufficient analgesia, consider prescribing acetaminophen combination drugs.[20] Acetaminophen include drugs like codeine, oxycodone, and hydrocodone in it.

Considerations for Nursing Mothers

Opioids pass into breast milk.[8] Prescribing opioids for a shorter period of time and using smaller doses provides the least risk for the nursing infant.[111]

Dental Analgesics

This section is intended to serve as a quick reference providing information to aid the clinician in determining what pain medications to use for the pregnant patient Prior to prescribing medication a risk-benefit analysis should always be done in in conjunction with the patient's prenatal care provider. In general, acetaminophen (plain) may be one of the safer medications.[22] When something stronger is needed, an acetaminophen combination drug may be considered.

Summary of select pain-management medications during pregnancy		
S.No.	**Drug**	**Comments**
1	Acetaminophen	If the patient has liver disease, the dose should be reduced OTC maximum labelled dose is 3 g/day
2	Celecoxib	Prophylactic if the patient has a sulfa drug allergy.
3	Acetaminophen + codeine	There is potential for hyper - or hypocodeine metabolism so it is suggested that its dose should be reduced it the patient has a liver disease
4	Ibuprofen	Avoid in late pregnancy
5	Hydrocodone + ibuprofen	Should not be used in the third trimester. Also, the dose may be reduced in patients with liver disease
6	Meperidine	Prolonged use is not recommended.
7	Hydrocodone + acetaminophen	Neonatal respiratory depression may occur so should be avoided shortly before delivery.
8	Oxycodone + acetaminophen	Not recommended around the time of labor and delivery. Reduced dosage for patients with liver disease
9	Hydromorphone	Contraindicated during labor and delivery

- **Aspirin (Acetylsalicylic Acid)**

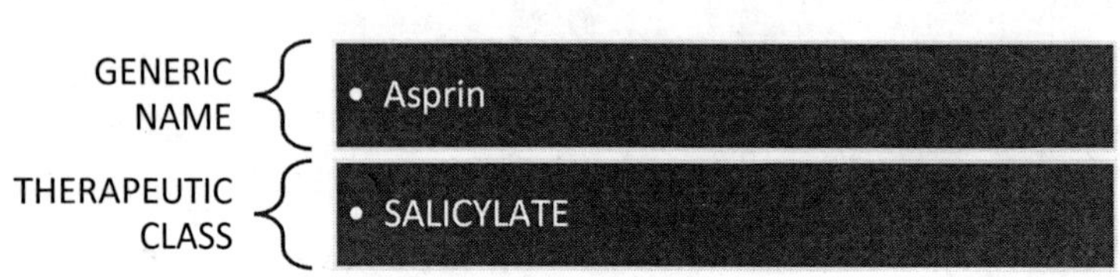

Pregnancy notes:

In general, aspirin-containing products should be avoided during pregnancy.[106] During the first two trimesters, aspirin is considered PRC C, but during the third trimester, it is considered PRC D.[20] Aspirin should be avoided in the first and third trimesters.[8,22] Physicians sometimes use low-dose aspirin to treat patients with certain medical conditions,such as antiphospholipid syndrome, during pregnancy.[136] Aspirin can cross to the fetus.[136] Aspirin inhibits prostaglandin synthesis and may cause the following:[8]

- Postponed labor and prolonged pregnancy[8]
- Delivery complications[8]
- Premature closure, or constriction, of the fetal ductus arteriosus, which may cause fetal pulmonary hypertension[20, 8]
- Antepartum maternal/fetal hemorrhage[20]
- Postpartum maternal/fetal hemorrhage[20]

Long-term aspirin use may be associated with maternal anemia.[20] High doses of aspirin may be associated with perinatal mortality, delayed intrauterine growth, and teratogenic effects.[20]

Aspirin may also be responsible for increased instances of spontaneous abortion or fetal gastroschisis (anterior abdominal wall defect that allows abdominal contents to protrude out).[111]

Risks with aspirin in the third trimester include low birth weight, increased incidence of intracranial hemorrhage in premature infants, stillbirth, neonatal death, anemia, and oligohydramnios (amniotic fluid deficiency).

If aspirin is taken within 1 week of labor and delivery, excessive blood loss may occur at delivery. Aspirin used several days before labor and delivery may cause intracranial hemorrhage in newborn infants.[8]

❖ Celecoxib

Celecoxib is a sulfa drug and is contraindicated for patients who are allergic to sulfa drugs.[133]

GENERIC NAME	• Celecoxib
THERAPEUTIC CLASS	• CELEBREX (Pfizer)

Pregnancy notes
Animal studies showed an increased incidence of the ventricular septal defect, diaphragmatic hernias when given celecoxib during organogenesis. Celecoxib should only be taken when the benefit to the patient is expected to outweigh the risk to the fetus.

Nursing notes
Celecoxib has been found to be excreted inhuman breast milk. The manufacturer recommends To use caution while administering to patients who are nursing.

Sample prescription
Rx: Celecoxib 200 mg **Disp:**15 capsules

❖ Ibuprofen

GENERIC NAME	• Ibuprofen
THERAPEUTIC CLASS	• ADVIL (Pfizer), MOTRIN (JOHNSON & JHONSON)

Pregnancy notes
Avoid using ibuprofen in the first and third trimesters, and avoid using ibuprofen for longer than 48 to 72 hours.[22] Ibuprofen is asked to be avoided in late pregnancy as it can cause premature closure of the ductus arteriosus.

Nursing notes
The manufacturer recommends against administering ibuprofen for patients who are nursing and advises that there is the potential for serious adverse reactions in infants who nurse from women taking ibuprofen.[135] **Note:** Others consider ibuprofen to be compatible with breastfeeding.

Sample prescription
Rx: Ibuprofen 600 mg **Disp:** 28 tablets **Sig:** Take 1 tablet by mouth every 8 hours, as needed for pain.[135] **Alternate sig:** Take 1tab po tid prn pain.

❖ Acetaminophen (N-acetyl-para-aminophenol)

Dosing may need to be reduced in patients with renal or hepatic impairment.[136] Consuming alcohol while taking acetaminophen increases the risk of developing hepatotoxicity.[136] Patients should be instructed to not take more than 3 g of acetaminophen per day unless directed by a health care professional who may recommend a maximum dose of 4 g per day.

GENERIC NAME	• Acetaminophen (N-acetyl-para-aminophenol or acetaminophen or paracetamol)
THERAPEUTIC CLASS	• Tylenol (Johnson & Johnson), Acephan (G&W Laboratories), Excedrin Tension Headache (GlaxoSmithKline), Mapap (Major Pharmaceuticals)

Pregnancy notes
Acetaminophen appears to be safe and has been widely used as an analgesic during pregnancy.[115] Some consider acetaminophen as the analgesic of choice for the short-term management of the pregnant patient's orofacial pain.[20,22] When given in high doses, it may be associated with maternal anemia and fetal renal disease.[8] Frequent use during pregnancy may be associated with early childhood asthma and wheezing.[136] Advise patients to make sure that the total acetaminophen from all sources does not exceed the maximum daily limit.[136]

Sample prescription
Rx: Acetaminophen **Disp:** (Available OTC) **Sig:** Take 325 to 650 mg by mouth every 4 to 6 hours. Do not exceed 4 g/day.[136] **Alternate sig:** Take 1,000 mg po tid. Do not exceed 4 g/day.

❖ **Acetaminophen + codeine**

This combination comes in two forms:

- Tylenol with Codeine #3 contains 300 mg of acetaminophen and 30 mg of codeine
- Tylenol with Codeine #4 contains 300 mg of acetaminophen and 60 mg of codeine

If the patient uses multiple medications that contain acetaminophen, she should be cautioned on the potential for acetaminophen overdose. Some people are ultra rapid metabolizers of codeine and are at risk of experiencing overdose symptoms.

GENERIC NAME	• acetaminophen + codeine
THERAPEUTIC CLASS	• Tylenol with Codeine

Pregnancy notes
Codeine passes to the fetus

Nursing notes
Both acetaminophen and codeine are excreted in human milk.

Sample prescription
Rx: Tylenol #3 **Disp:** 28 tablets **Sig:** Take 1 to 2 tablets by mouth every 4 to 6 hours as needed for pain.

❖ **Aspirin + caffeine + dihydrocodeine**

GENERIC NAME	• Aspirin + caffeine + dihydrocodeine
THERAPEUTIC CLASS	• Synalgos-DC (Sun Pharmaceutical Industries)

Pregnancy note
There is currently insufficient information to know the possible adverse fetal effects. codeine may be associated with multiple congenital defects that include heart and circulatory defects, cleft lip, and cleft palate.[21]

Nursing notes
It is not recommended in nursing mothers unless the benefit clearly outweighs the risks. Infant death may occur when infants are exposed to larger-than-usual amounts of morphine in the breast milk of mothers who are rapid metabolizers of codeine.

Ingredients
Aspirin (356.4 mg) Caffeine (30 mg) Dihydrocodeine (16 mg)

- **Tramadol + acetaminophen**

GENERIC NAME	• Tramadol + acetaminophen
THERAPEUTIC CLASS	• Ultracet (Janssen Pharmaceuticals)

Pregnancy notes
Acetaminophen and tramadol both cross to the placenta.[136] Tramadol has been reported to be possibly linked with neonatal seizures, neonatal withdrawal syndrome, fetal death, and stillbirth.[136]

Nursing notes
It is not recommended for nursing mothers to use Ultracet in nursing mothers as its safety has not been studied. One study showed that 16 hours after a single maternal IV dose of tramadol, 0.1 % of the maternal dose was present in human breast milk.

Active ingredients
Acetaminophen (325 mg) Tramadol hydrochloride (37.5 mg)

❖ Hydrocodone + acetaminophen

GENERIC NAME
- Hydrocodone + acetaminophen

THERAPEUTIC CLASS
- Norco, Lorcet (Forest Pharmaceuticals), Lortab
- (Akorn, Inc), Vicodin

Pregnancy notes
Use may lead to fetal physical dependency and neonatal withdrawal symptoms at delivery.[136] The intensity does not always correlate with maternal duration or dose. Neonatal respiratory depression can be caused if Vicodin is given to the expectant mother shortly before delivery.

Nursing notes
Acetaminophen is excreted in human breast Milk.[136] Because of the limited studies and the possibility of serious adverse reactions in the nursing infant, nursing is not recommended while the mother is taking hydrocodone +acetaminophen.

Nursing notes
Acetaminophen is excreted in human breast Milk.[136] Because of the limited studies and the possibility of serious adverse reactions in the nursing infant, nursing is not recommended while the mother is taking hydrocodone +acetaminophen.

Sample prescription
Rx: Vicodin (5 mg/300 mg) **Disp:** 16 tablets **Alternate sig:** Take 1–2 tabs 4–6h prn pain, not to exceed 8 tabs in 24 hours.

❖ Hydrocodone + ibuprofen

GENERIC NAME
- Hydrocodone + ibuprofen

THERAPEUTIC CLASS
- Ibudone (Poly Pharmaceuticals),
- Vicoprofen (AbbVie)

Pregnancy notes
It may lead to the fetal ductus arteriosus prematurely closing hence Vicoprofen should not be used in late pregnancy (third trimester).

Nursing notes
Because of the limited studies and the possibility of serious adverse reactions in the nursing infant, nursing is not recommended while the mother is taking Vicoprofen.

Sample prescription
Rx: Vicoprofen **Disp:** 16 tablets **Sig:** Take 1 tablet by mouth every 4 to 6 hours as needed for pain. Do not exceed 5 tablets in 24 hours.

❖ Oxycodone + aspirin

GENERIC NAME	• Oxycodone + aspirin
THERAPEUTIC CLASS	• Endodan (Endo Pharmaceuticals), Percodan • (Endo Pharmaceuticals)

Pregnancy notes

Oxycodone has not been found to be teratogenic or toxic to the fetus in rat and rabbit studies. Neonatal respiratory depression can be caused to the fetus as oxycodone can cross to it. fetal physical drug dependency, and withdrawal symptoms after birth can also be seen. Percodan is not recommended just prior to labor and delivery because it may depress the newborn respiratory system.[136]

Nursing notes

Because of the risk of adverse reactions to the nursing infant, the mother should normally either discontinue nursing or discontinue the use of this drug[136] sedation and respiratory depression can be caused in the nursing infant as Oxycodone is found in human breast milk. There have been reports of somnolence and lethargy in babies of nursing mothers who have been taking an oxycodone/acetaminophen combination drug.

Aspirin has been detected in human breastmilk. The nursing infant is at increased risk for problems with platelet functioning. The nursing infant is also at increased risk for getting Reye syndrome (acute brain damage and liver dysfunction).

❖ Oxycodone + acetaminophen

Percocet (Endo Pharmaceuticals) comes in several different strengths

GENERIC NAME	• Oxycodone + acetaminophen
THERAPEUTIC CLASS	• Percocet

Pregnancy notes
Neonatal respiratory depression can be caused as a result of opioids as it can cross to fetus. Fetal exposure to opioids may cause the neonate to suffer symptoms of severe drug withdrawal,which may be life-threatening.[136] This drug is not recommended for use by women around the time of labor and delivery because it may lead to depressed respiratory function of the newborn.

Nursing notes
Small amounts of both acetaminophen and oxycodone have been found in human breast milk.There have been reports of somnolence and lethargy in babies of nursing mothers who have been taking an oxycodone/acetaminophen combination drug. The nursing infant is at risk of sedation and respiratory depression.

Sample prescription
Rx: Percocet 2.5 mg **Disp:** 20 tablets **Alternate sig**: Take 1–2 tabs po q6h prn pain.

❖ **Meperidine**

GENERIC NAME	• Meperidine
THERAPEUTIC CLASS	• Demerol (Pfizer)

Pregnancy notes
While meperidine may be used in pregnancy,prolonged use of meperidine is not recommended.[22,124] Meperidine has not been studied in animal reproductive studies. Meperidine crosses the placenta and accumulates in the fetus, and it should not be used around the time of labor and delivery because it can travel from the pregnant woman to the fetus, where it may depress respiratory and psychophysiological functions.[136] The newborn infant may require resuscitation.

Nursing notes
Meperidine can be found in human breastmilk. This may place the nursing infant at risk for serious adverse reactions. a nursing mother should either discontinue using or switch medications.[8]

Sample prescription
Rx: Demerol 50 mg **Disp**: 16 tablets.

❖ **Hydromorphone**

GENERIC NAME
- Hydromorphone

THERAPEUTIC CLASS
- Dilaudid (Fresenius Kabi)

Pregnancy notes
Hydromorphone crosses the placenta and is present in the fetus. Animal studies show increased incidence of exencephaly (cephalic disorder where brain tissue protrudes outside of the skull) and cranioschisis (failure of the skull to completely fuse) when given during organogenesis. Dilaudid is contraindicate during labor and delivery.

Nursing notes
Nursing should be discontinued while the mother is taking this medication as it can be present in the mothers milk.

Sample prescription
Rx: Dilaudid 2 mg **Disp:** 16 tablets **Sig:** Take 1 tablet by mouth every 4 to 6 hours as needed for pain.

Dental Antibiotics

This section is intended to serve as a quick reference, providing information to aid the clinician in determining what antibiotic to use for the pregnant patient. It is important to be aware that some antibiotics have altered pharmacokinetics during pregnancy.This may cause changes in drug effectiveness during pregnancy.

Families of Antibiotics commonly used in Dentistry

Family: Penicillins
• **Action:** Inhibits bacterial cell wall synthesis[137] • Comments **Example:** **i)** Penicillin **ii)** Amoxicillin **iii)** Oxacillin **iv)** Cloxacillin **v)** Dicloxacillin **vi)** Methicillin **vii)** Ampicillin

Family: Cephalosporins
• **Action:** Inhibits bacterial cell wall synthesis.[137] • Comments **1. First-generation:** **i)** Cefazolin **ii)** Cephalexin **iii)** Cefadroxil **iv)** Cefradine **v)** Second generation **vi)** Cefuroxime **vii)** Cefprozil **viii)** Cefmetazole

Family: Macrolides
• **Action:** Acts on the 50S ribosomal subunit, which inhibits tRNAtranslocation[137] • **Comments:** **Examples:** • Erythromycin • Clarithromycin • Roxithromycin • Azithromycin1 Macrolide antibiotics may cause a prolonged QT interval (irregular heart rhythm).[136]

Family: Tetracyclines
• **Action:** Bacteriostatic: Binds ribosomal30S subunit, inhibiting RNA aminoacyl transferase137 • **Comments** **Examples:** Tetracycline and doxycycline, which are PRC D Tetracyclines have been linked to dental developmental problems such as staining and hypomineralization. Tetracyclines should be avoided during pregnancy and also in nursing mothers.[8,137]

Family: Lincosamines
• **Action:** Acts on the 50S ribosomal subunit to inhibit tRNA translocation. • **Comments:** **Examples:** Clindamycin is the only lincosamine indicated for pregnant women.[130]

Family: Quinolones
• **Action:** Converts bacterial gyrase and topoisomerase IV into toxic enzymes that fragment the bacterial chromosome.[138] • **Comments:** **Example:** ciprofloxacin[139] Quinolones act via a different mechanism than penicillins, cephalosporins, aminoglycosides, macrolides, and tetracyclines.[139] Microorganisms resistant to these classes of antibiotics may be susceptible to quinolones.[139] There is no known cross-resistance between ciprofloxacin and other antimicrobial classes.

Antibiotics commonly used in dentistry:

- **Penicillin V potassium:** May require higher dose or increased dosing frequency during second and third trimesters.
- **Amoxicillin:** Decreased peak serum concentration and decreased half-life during pregnancy.
- **Amoxicillin + clavulanic acid:** Decreased peak serum concentration and decreased half-life during pregnancy. Not recommended for use in women with preterm premature rupture of fetal membrane.
- **Dicloxacillin:** Animal studies have not shown harm to the fetus.
- **Cephalexin:** Pregnancy does not appear to alter peak concentrations of cephalexin.
- **Clarithromycin:** PRC C. Inform pregnant patients of potential harm to the fetus.
- **Erythromycin:** Avoid the estolate form. This drug has multiple drug interactions.
- **Azithromycin:** Azithromycin may lead to irregular heart rhythm in the a patient that can be fatal.
- **Clindamycin:** Pregnancy does not appear to alter the pharmacokinetics.
- **Ciprofloxacin:** PRC C. Teratogenic risk is unlikely, but clindamycin should be reserved for patients with no other treatment options.

Penicillin V Potassium

GENERIC NAME: Penicillin V potassium

Antibiotic family: Penicillins

Pregnancy notes
It can cross the placenta entering the amniotic fluid. Maternal penicillin use is generally thought to be safe and does not increase the risk of adverse fetal effects,[133] the pharmacokinetics of penicillin may be altered during the second and third trimesters of pregnancy. This may require the use of a larger dose or increased dosing frequency to obtain the same effect. A study has suggested to increase the dosage frequency to every 6 hours (q6h)

Nursing notes
Infants have been reported to have loose stools and rash after nursing from women who have taken penicillin.[136]

Sample prescription
Rx: Penicillin V potassium 500 mg
Disp: 40 tablets
Sig: Take 1 tablet by mouth 4 times per day until gone.[140]

❖ Amoxicillin

GENERIC NAME: Amoxicillin

Antibiotic family: Penicillins

Pregnancy notes
In general, maternal amoxicillin use has not shown an increased risk of adverse fetal effects.[141] Maternal exposure to amoxicillin may increase fetal risk of cleft lip or cleft palate.[140] Pregnancy-induced physiologic changes include increased clearance due to: • Decreased peak (maximum) serum concentration (Cmax) • Decreased amoxicillin half-life

Nursing notes
The manufacturer recommends caution when using amoxicillin in mothers who are nursing[140]. As the amoxicillin has been found in breast milk it may lead to infant allergic sensitization or even a risk of altering infant bowel flora.

Sample prescription
Rx: Amoxicillin 500 mg **Disp:** 30 tablets **Sig:** Take 1 tablet by mouth 3 times per day until gone.[142]

❖ **Amoxicillin + clavulanic acid**

GENERIC NAME { • Amoxicillin + clavulanic acid

Antibiotic family { • Penicillins

Pregnancy notes
Augmentin may be associated with increased risk of bowel disorders such as neonatal necrotizing enterocolitis. It is not recommended for use in women with preterm premature rupture of fetal membrane, as it may be associated with increased risk of neonatal necrotizing entercolitis.

Nursing notes
Amoxicillin is present in human breast milk. The manufacturer recommends caution in Nursing

Sample prescription
Rx: Augmentin 500 mg **Disp:** 30 tablets

- **Dicloxacillin**

GENERIC NAME: • Dicloxacillin

Antibiotic family: • Penicillins

Pregnancy notes
Small amounts of dicloxacillin have been found to cross from the pregnant woman to the fetus during late pregnancy, but animal studies have not shown harm to the fetus.[143]

Nursing notes
The manufacturer recommends caution when using dicloxacillin in nursing mothers.[143] Other penicillins are excreted in human milk and are considered safe during breastfeeding There is a risk of altering infant bowel flora.

Sample prescription
Rx: Dicloxacillin 500 mg **Disp**: 40 capsules

❖ Cephalexin

GENERIC NAME	• Cephalexin
Antibiotic family	• Cephalosporins

Pregnancy notes
Maternal cephalexin can be found at therapeutic levels in amniotic fluid and in the fetal circulation.[136] Cephalexin has not been associated with an increased risk of teratogenic events.[142]

Nursing notes
The manufacturer recommends caution when using dicloxacillin in nursing mothers.[143] Other penicillins are excreted in human milk and are considered safe during breastfeeding. There is a risk of altering infant bowel flora.

Sample prescription
Rx: Cephalexin 500 mg
Disp: 40 capsules
Sig: Take 1 capsule by mouth 4 times per day until gone.[136]

❖ Clarithromycin

GENERIC NAME	• Clarithromycin
Antibiotic family	• Macrolides

Pregnancy notes
Animal studies have shown adverse fetal effects. The manufacturer recommends that clarithromycin should only be used in pregnant women when there is no appropriate alternative therapy.[142] If pregnancy occurs while the patient is taking clarithromycin, the manufacturer recommends informing the patient of the possible harm to the fetus

Nursing notes
The manufacturer recommends caution if administering clarithromycin to a nursing woman.[136] Clarithromycin is excreted in human milk.[142]

Additional warnings
Clarithromycin may cause a prolonged QT interval (irregular heart rhythm).[136]

❖ **Erythromycin**

GENERIC NAME	• Erythromycin
Antibiotic family	• Macrolides

Pregnancy notes
Erythromycin crosses to the placenta.[136] Adverse effects include abdominal pain.[136] The enteric coating may decrease the risk of causing an upset stomach.[136] Avoid the estolate form during pregnancy and breastfeeding.[137,133] The estolate form may be more hepatotoxic during pregnancy than the non estolate form.[133] The estolate form is associated with cholestatic hepatitis during pregnancy.[70]

Nursing notes
Erythromycin is excreted in human breastmilk, so use caution in nursing.

Sample prescription
Rx: Erythromycin base 250 mg **Disp:** 40 tablets (enteric coated) **Sig:** Take 1 tablet by mouth 4 times per day until gone.[70]

Additional warnings
Multiple drug interactions and fatalities have been reported. When prescribing, refer to an up-to-date drug reference for further information. Erythromycin may cause irregular heart rhythm..

- **Azithromycin**

GENERIC NAME	• Azithromycin
Antibiotic family	• Macrolides

Pregnancy notes
When compared with other antibiotics, azithromycin does not cross the placenta to the fetus as easily.[115] It is recommend for use in pregnant women who are allergic to penicillin.[113] Limited information suggests that azithromycin may be a cause for infantile pyloric stenosis, which is the narrowing of the opening that goes from the stomach to the duodenum. The serum half-life of azithromycin is not affected in early pregnancy; at term, serum half-life is decreased. After 48 hours, concentrations were found to be similar. High concentrations of azithromycin are present in the myometrium (uterine wall's middle layer) and also adipose tissue.

Nursing notes
The manufacturer recommends caution during nursing.[136] Azithromycin is excreted in human breast milk. Altered bowel flora, diarrhea, rash, somnolence, and decreased appetite have been reported in nursing infants.

Sample prescription
Note: Zithromax is packaged in a Z-Pak.
Rx: Zithromax (Z-Pak)
Disp: 1 pack (6 × 250 mg tablets)
Sig: Take 2 tablets by mouth on day 1, and 1 tablet on days 2 through 5.[47]

- **Clindamycin**

GENERIC NAME: • Clindamycin

Antibiotic family: • Lincosamides

Pregnancy notes
Clindamycin crosses the placenta to the fetus. Maternal use of clindamycin has not been associated with adverse fetal effects.[144]
The pharmacokinetics do not appear to be altered during pregnancy.[136]

Nursing notes
Clindamycin is excreted in human breastmilk.[144] While some authors suggest that clindamycin is safe for use during breastfeeding, the manufacturer recommends against using clindamycin for nursing mothers.[111]

Sample prescription
Rx: Clindamycin 300 mg
Disp: 40 capsules
Sig: Take 1 capsule by mouth 4 times per day until gone.[144]

Additional warnings
Multiple drug interactions and fatalities have been reported. When prescribing, refer to an up-to-date drug reference for further information. Erythromycin may cause a irregular heart rhythm.

❖ Ciprofloxacin

GENERIC NAME: • Ciprofloxacin

Antibiotic family: • Quinolones

Pregnancy notes
An expert review of published data concluded that it is unlikely that substantial teratogenic risk exists when therapeutic doses of ciprofloxacin are taken during pregnancy.[139] Several small postmarketing epidemiologic studies suggest that ciprofloxacin is safe during pregnancy. To confirm these initial findings more research has to be conducted. Animal studies have shown that quinolones (including ciprofloxacin) cause arthropathy in weight-bearing joints in juveniles, resulting in lameness.

Nursing notes
Ciprofloxacin is excreted in human breast milk.[139] The manufacturer recommends against breast feeding while the mother is taking ciprofloxacin.

Additional warning
Excerpt from a 2016 FDA safety announcement: "We have determined that fluoroquinolones should be reserved for use in patients who have no other treatment options because the risk of these serious side effects generally outweighs the benefits in these patients. For some serious bacterial infections, the benefits of fluoroquinolones outweigh the risks, and it is appropriate for them to remain available as a therapeutic option. Stop fluoroquinolone treatment immediately if a patient reports serious side effects, and switch to a non-fluoroquinolone antibacterial drug to complete the patient's treatment course.[144]"

FDA classification of drug therapy for gastroesophageal reflux disease in pregnancy[142]

1. **Antacids**
    - Aluminum-containing antacids
    - Calcium-containing antacids
    - Magnesium-containingantacids
2. **Magnesium trisilicates**
3. **Sodium bicarbonate**
4. **Mucosal protectant Sucralfate**
5. **H2RAs**
6. **Cimetidine**
7. **Ranitidine**
8. **Famotidine**
9. **Nizatidine**
10. **Cisapride**
11. **Metoclopramide**
12. **Proton pump inhibitors Omeprazole**
13. **Lansoprazole**
14. **Rabeprazole**
15. **Pantoprazole**
16. **Esomeprazole**

Pregnancy and Heartburn

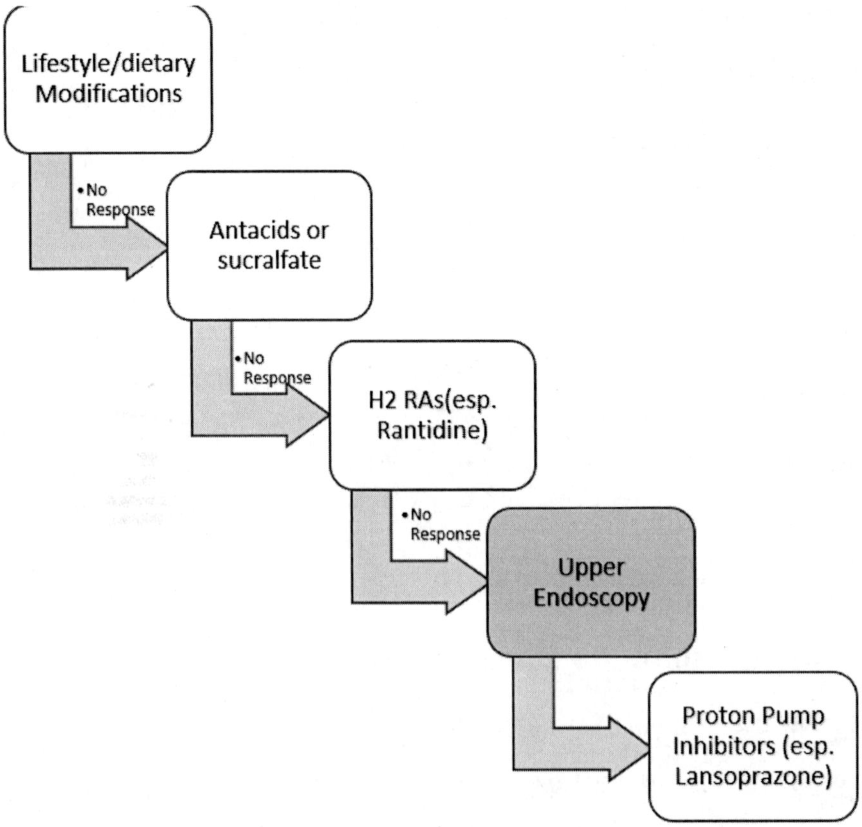

Anesthetic Use

Common dental topical anesthetics:

1. Topical:

- Lidocaine
- Lidocaine and prilocaine combination (eg, Oraqix)
- Benzocaine
- Tetracaine
- Benzocaine/butamben/tetracaine combination

2. Local:

- Articaine
- Bupivacaine
- Lidocaine with or without epinephrine
- Mepivacaine
- Prilocaine

Calculating the Amount of Local Anesthetic in a Dental Cartridge

The American Academy of Pediatric Dentistry recommends using 1.8 when calculating the maximum dosage of local anesthetic for all patients.For every 100 ml of a solution that contains 2% local anesthetic, there are 2 g (2,000 mg)local anesthetic.[9] With this ratio of 20 mg/ml, the amount of anesthetic in a 1.8-mL dental cartridge can be calculated as 36 mg.[145]

$$2\%\ \text{anesthetic} = \frac{2\ \text{g anesthetic}}{100\ \text{mL}} = \frac{2{,}000\ \text{mg anesthetic}}{100\ \text{mL}} = \frac{20\ \text{mg anesthetic}}{1\ \text{mL}}$$

$$\frac{20\ \text{mg anesthetic}}{1\ \text{mL}} \times \frac{1.8\ \text{ml}}{\text{dental cartridge}} = \frac{36\ \text{mg anesthetic}}{\text{dental cartridge}}$$

Allergies and Psychogenic Reactions

Local and topical anesthetics can be divided into the categories of esters and amides based on their molecular structure.[146] While topical amide and ester anesthetics are available, only amide local dental anesthetic cartridges are available in the United States. Because most allergic reactions to local anesthetics are to ester anesthetic, not amide, it is more likely that the patient will be allergic to a topical anesthetic than a local anesthetic.[21] The suspected allergen in ester anesthetics is the metabolite para-aminobenzoic acid.[21] Articaine has an ester linkage;however, it quickly breaks down into an inactive metabolite.[21] Dental anesthetic cartridges may contain compounds such as epinephrine orlevonordefrin (eg, Neo-Cobefrin, Cook-Waite), which are vasoconstrictors. If a vasoconstrictor is present, the dental anesthetic cartridge will also include an antioxidant.[21] The antioxidant can be sodium bisulfite or metabisulfite. A bisulfite allergy is thought to be much more common than a true allergy to the local anesthetic.[21]

It is estimated that 59% to 77% of adverse reactions to local anesthetics are due to psychogenic causes.[147] Symptoms of psychogenic reactions may include dizziness, pallor, nausea, palpitations, fainting, vasovagal syncope, and other autonomic responses. Psychogenic reactions usually begin within 1 to 2 minutes of administration of the local anesthetic. Other less common causes of adverse reactions include allergy and inadvertent intravascular injection.[147]

Effect on Dental Treatment

The most common cause of an adverse reaction to a local or topical anesthetic is a psychogenic reaction.[148] If it is suspected that a patient may have a true allergy to an anesthetic, the patient can be referred for allergy testing prior to treatment.[21]

Lists Which Anesthetic Might Be Considered If the Patient Has an Allergy

Dental anesthetic allergies and solutions[21]

S.No.	Allergic to	Alternative
1.	Ester anesthetics	Amide anesthetic
2.	Amide anesthetic	Ester anesthetic
3.	Antioxidant (sodium bisulfite or metabisulfite)	Anesthetic free of antioxidant. (Because this antioxidant is added when a vasoconstrictor is added, these anesthetics will have no vasoconstrictor.)

Methemoglobinemia

Methemoglobinemia occurs when the oxidation state of iron in the hemoglobin molecule changes from Fe^{2+} (ferrous state) to Fe^{3+} (ferric state).[146] This prevents hemoglobin from transporting oxygen.[149] Depending on the severity, the patient may exhibit arange of symptoms of lack of oxygen and respiratory distress.[146] Symptoms are not relieved with the administration of 100% oxygen because not all hemoglobin molecules are properly functioning. Methemoglobinemia is often treated by methylene blue.While rare, methemoglobinemia can lead to death.[146]

Effect on Dental Treatment

Certain topical and local anesthetics used in dentistry may increase the risk for acquired methemoglobinemia.[149] Because symptoms may occur 3 to 4 hours after exposure, the patient may no longer be in the dental office.[146]

Topical Anesthetics

This section is intended to serve as a quick reference providing information to aid the clinician in determining what topical anesthetic(s) to use. It is intended to be used as a starting point, not to replace an up-to-date drug reference or the clinical judgment of licensed health care professionals.

❖ Lidocaine (topical)

GENERIC NAME { • Lidocaine (topical)

Pregnancy notes
No evidence of fetal harm has been observed in studies with rats at up to 6.6 times the recommended human dose.[150,148].

Nursing notes
Unknown if excreted in human breast milk. Lidocaine is thought to be safe for the nursing Infant.[150,148]

Additional warning
In children under 3 years of age, cardiopulmonary arrest and death may occur when not used in accordance with recommended dosage and administration.[150,148]

❖ Lidocaine + prilocaine combination

GENERIC NAME { • Lidocaine + prilocaine combination

Pregnancy notes
The combination of lidocaine and prilocaine (eg,Oraqix)[151] show no fetal harm

Nursing notes
May be excreted in human breast milk. The manufacturer recommends caution when administering to mothers who are nursing.[151] Based on separate entries, the LactMed database indicates that dental topical application of lidocaine and prilocaine is unlikely to affect the nursing infant.

Additional warning
Lidocaine and prilocaine toxicities are thought to be additive.[151] It should be avoided in patients who have a history of congenital or acquired methemoglobinemia.

- **Benzocaine**

GENERIC NAME { • Benzocaine

Pregnancy notes
Benzocaine is sometimes recommended as a topical anesthetic that is safe to use during pregnancy. Fetal complications have not been observed in the limited studies that have included benzocaine as a topical anesthetic.[21] When choosing a topical anesthetic,the practitioner should be aware that benzocaineis FDA PRC C and that PRC B topical anesthetics are available.

Nursing notes
Maternal dental topical application is unlikely to have a negative effect on the nursing infant.[147]

- **Tetracaine**

GENERIC NAME { • Tetracaine

Pregnancy notes
Caution is advised when using tetracaine on the pregnant patient.[111]

Nursing notes
Maternal dental topical application is unlikely to have a negative effect on the nursing infant.[147]

❖ **Benzocaine/butamben/tetracaine**

GENERIC NAME { • Benzocaine/butamben/tetracaine

Pregnancy notes
It is not known if this combination of topical anesthetics may have adverse fetal effects.[149]

Nursing notes
Benzocaine: It is not likely to have a negative effect on the nursing infant due to maternal dental topical application. **Butamben:** There has not been sufficient research on the effect of maternal use on the nursing infant. **Tetracaine:** Maternal dental topical application is unlikely to have a negative effect on the nursing infant.

Additional warning
Benzocaine and tetracaine should be avoided in patients with a history of congenital or acquired methemoglobinemia.[138]

Local Anesthetics

Fetal Exposure to Local Anesthetics During Pregnancy

Local anesthetic administered to a pregnant woman also freely passes to the Fetus.[8,115,21,133] Fetal toxicity depends on the amount of anesthetic that the fetus receives.[21] The amount of local anesthetic reaching the fetus is usually thought to be insufficient to create an adverse reaction.

Factors that appear to affect the passage of local anesthetic from the patient to the fetus include the following:[21]

- Administration route eg, intramuscular, accidental intravascular
- Presence or absence of a vasoconstrictor
- Maternal protein binding
- Fetal protein binding

Local anesthetics without a vasoconstrictor have been shown to affect uterine smooth muscle.[21] In vitro studies have indicated that large amounts of lidocaine can result in contractions. However, these adverse effects have not been observed in vivo when using clinically acceptable amounts of lidocaine.[21]

Amide local anesthetics require 1-acid glycoprotein for metabolism, and during pregnancy, there is a decreased amount of 1-acid glycoprotein.[8,21] This indicates that it is more likely that a pregnant women will have more plasma-free local anesthetic after administration. In turn, the fetus will be exposed to more local anesthetic, which increases the risk of fetal toxicity.[8,21] Because of this increased possibility of local anesthetic toxicity during pregnancy, consider administering a reduced dose to pregnant women.[8,21]

Effect on Dental Treatment

Local anesthetics administered to the pregnant patient can cross to the fetus, where they may lead to fetal depression.[133] Care should also be taken to avoid accidental intravascular injection, which may cause complications such as convulsions, coma,and respiratory arrest.[21,111,123] In the presence of certain medical conditions such as preeclampsia or eclampsia, inadvertent intravascular injection increases the possibility of inducing a seizure.[21] Avoid longer-acting anesthetics such as bupivacaine if a shorter-acting anesthetic would be adequate, because longer-acting anesthetics may provide greater risk to the fetus.[8,21,111]

As with most medications, lidocaine has not undergone adequate well-controlled studies in pregnant women to establish safe use during pregnancy.[152] However, based on its track record, lidocaine with epinephrine may be the anesthetic of choice during pregnancy.[21] Epinephrine is thought to be a safer vasoconstrictor for the fetus when compared with levonordefrin.[21] Lidocaine with epinephrine is considered safe to use when providing necessary dental treatment during pregnancy.[113,117] To minimize possible fetal risk, it is recommended to use the minimum effective dose of local anesthetic.[154] It has been recommended to proportionally reduce the maximum dosage of local anesthetics as its toxicity may be higher in pregnancy.

Local Anesthetic Use During the Immediate Postpartum Period

During the immediate postpartum period (at least the first 2 to 3 weeks after delivery),the patient will often be in a hypercoagulable state. Some studies suggest that the condition can last for up to 25 days after delivery, and possibly longer.[21] Because of the hypercoagulable state, the perinatal care provider may prescribe prophylactic anticoagulation medication. Epinephrine may also worsen the hypercoagulable state.

Epinephrine may activate coagulation by increasing thrombin and clotting factor VIII levels. The amount of epinephrine from the local anesthetic is thought to be minimal during normal intramuscular injections. However, an accidental intravascular injection may have the potential to introduce a significant amount of epinephrine.[21]

Effect on Dental Treatment

Because the woman may be in a hypercoagulable state, consider if the need to provide dental treatment is urgent or if the patient can wait a few weeks. Use good local anesthetic administration technique, including aspiration to minimize accidental intravascular injection.[8,20,21]

Local Anesthetic Use During Lactation

While a true allergy to lidocaine is rare, adding epinephrine as a vasoconstrictor requires the addition of preservatives to the dental cartridge.[21] During lactation, an infant can have an adverse reaction to these preservatives.[21]

Effect on Dental Treatment

Be aware of the possibility that a nursing infant may have an adverse reaction to a local anesthetic administered to the mother.[21] If there is a concern that a significant amount of the drug might be passed on to the infant, consider suggesting that feeding be accomplished with stored milk or formula. The shorter the half-life of the medication,the sooner the mother can return to nursing her child.

Local Anesthetic Quick Guide

This section is intended to serve as a quick reference providing information to aid the clinician in determining what local anesthetic(s) to use for the pregnant patient. It is not intended to replace an up-to-date drug reference, which should be consulted when prescribing any medication. Please see the following sections for the maximum recommended dosages of individual anesthetics for pregnant patients.

❖ **Lidocaine**

GENERIC NAME
• Lidocaine

Pregnancy notes
Inadvertent intravascular injection may expose the fetus or uterus to significant levels of epinephrine.[45] Lidocaine is the local anesthetic with the longest track record and is the most commonly used local anesthetic.

Nursing notes
The manufacturer recommends caution and states that it is unknown if lidocaine is present in human breast milk. The American Academy of Pediatrics considers lidocaine to be safe for breastfeeding mothers.[21]

❖ Mepivacaine

GENERIC NAME
- Mepivacaine

Pregnancy notes
Risk of fetal bradycardia (decreased fetal heart rate).[20,153] Epinephrine is thought to be a safer vasoconstrictor for the fetus than levonordefrin.[21]

Nursing notes
It is unknown whether mepivacaine is present in human breast milk or not so caution should be taken

❖ Prilocaine

GENERIC NAME
- Prilocaine

Pregnancy notes
Possible risk of fetal methemoglobinemia.

Nursing notes
Unknown if found in human breast milk.

Additional warning
Prilocaine should be avoided in patients with a history of congenital or acquired methemglobinemia.

❖ **Bupivacaine**

GENERIC NAME – • Bupivacaine

Pregnancy notes
Risk of fetal bradycardia.[20] May have an increased risk of fetal toxicity when compared with other shorter-acting local anesthetics.[8]

Nursing notes
Unknown if present in human breast milk.

Additional warning
Bupivacaine is not recommended for children under 12 years.[152,154]

❖ **Articaine**

GENERIC NAME – Articaine

Pregnancy notes
Animal studies show the risk of fetal harm.Only use during pregnancy if the benefit will likely outweigh the fetal risk. Safe use on children under the age of 4 years has not been established.

Nursing notes
Unknown if present in human breast milk.Safe use on children under the age of 4 years has not been established. To minimize the chance of this drug getting to the infant,nursing mothers may pump and discard breast milk for 4 hours (based on the plasma half-life).

Nitrous Oxide

Use of nitrous oxide in pregnant women is a controversial topic. Nitrous oxide can travel to the placenta and may interfere with DNA synthesis or cause vasoconstriction, decreasing uterine blood flow.[20,155] The use of nitrous oxide has also been implicated in spontaneous abortion in women with occupational exposure. Because of potential contraindications, nitrous oxide use is restricted to situations where local and topical anesthesia are insufficient to provide treatment that is both necessary and non deferrable. When used alone, nitrous oxide has an excellent safety record.[22] As a single agent, nitrous oxide does not depress ventilation.[22] When combined with other medications that depress ventilation (eg, sedatives or opioids), a greater-than-expected respiratory depression may occur.[22] Consider treating pregnant women who require sedation with general anesthesia in a hospital.[113]

Effect on Dental Treatment

Nitrous oxide has a greater effect on pregnant women than non-pregnant women. It takes a lower dosage of nitrous oxide to have the same effect.[22,113,117] If possible, avoid using nitrous oxide during the first trimester.[21,8,20,106] If nitrous oxide is administered, it will ideally be in the second or third trimester and administered with at least 50% oxygen and for less than 30 minutes.[8,123]

Avoid prolonged treatments with nitrous oxide to minimize fetal exposure to nitrous oxide.[22] Use standard nitrous oxide administration protocols in dentistry, and continuously monitor vital signs when administering nitrous oxide.[22] Use a scavenging system to minimize gas escape and indirect exposure to nitrous oxide during administration.[22,123]

Maintenance of Good Oral Health During Pregnancy

At-Home Oral Care

Dental treatment is only one piece of the patient's overall oral health. For the pregnant women to take an active role in maintaining their oral health,it is important to teach them how to take care of their oral hygiene at home. It is important to provide oral hygiene instructions and explain how diet affects oral health as a part of educating the patient about at home oral care. Because of the oral changes that occur during pregnancy, including the increased prevalence of gingivitis, it is especially important for the patient to maintain meticulous oral hygiene throughout her pregnancy, Brushing, flossing, and mouthwash.

Toothbrush Instructions

Each person in a family should have his or her own toothbrush, and toothbrushes should not be shared[145]. Toothbrushes should be replaced at the first sign of wear, or every 3 to 4 months. Toothbrushes with soft bristles should be chosen.[105]

Toothpaste Selection

In order to aid in the removal of plaque and bacterial biofilm Toothpaste, or dentifrice is designed, this can be achieved by improving the mechanical cleaning that a toothbrush can provide. ADA seal of acceptance is more rigorous than the FDA's requirements for those manufacturing toothpaste. In addition to the mild abrasive that toothpastes typically contain, they may contain a number of other ingredients depending on the purpose of the toothpaste. Pyrophosphates, triclosan, or zinc citrate are the ingredients that may be found in toothpastes that reduces accumulation of calculus. A stain-removing toothpaste may have abrasives that are made of modified silica abrasives or enzymes.[155]

Brushing Technique

Some general recommendations can be used as a starting point besides using specific brushing technique for the specific patient. All patients should brush their teeth at least twice a day for 2 minutes.[155] It is particularly important for them to brush their teeth and use dental floss before going to bed.[22] They should use a toothpaste that contains fluoride, brush with gentle pressure, and position the toothbrush at a 45-degree angle to the gums and the teeth.[126] It is important to brush the outer, inner, and occlusal surfaces of the teeth as well as the gingival sulcus. In addition, patients should also brush their tongue to remove bacteria.

Use of Interdental Cleaners

In general, patients should use an interdental cleaner such as dental floss at least once a day.[124,22,113] According to specific needs of the individual patient the appropriate inter-dental cleaner and the proper technique should be selected.

Use of Mouthwash

In addition to brushing and flossing, patients should also use mouthwash.[118] By rinsing with a fluoride-containing alcohol-free mouth rinse right before going to bed, patients can help to remineralize their teeth.[124]

Oral Care After Vomiting

Vomiting increases acidity in the mouth and also places digestive enzymes (pepsin and trypsin) in the oral cavity, which may transiently increase the risk for tooth demineralization and erosion.[109] The patient should avoid brushing for about 1 hour after vomiting because brushing teeth immediately after vomiting can worsen tooth demineralization.[22,118,123]

To help neutralize acidity and minimize dental erosion, the woman should do one of the following immediately after vomiting:

- Rinse with water.
- Rinse with water with baking soda (sodium bicarbonate). Use an 8 oz cup of water that contain 1 tsp of baking soda.
- Rinse with a fluoride-containing mouthwash.
- Apply or gently brush casein phosphopeptide amorphous calcium phosphatepaste (eg, MI Paste) onto the teeth.

Nutritional Counseling

Eating healthy is good for both the patient's body and her teeth.

1. Eat Healthy Foods

Pregnant patients should be encouraged to eat a variety of healthy foods such as fruits, vegetables, whole-grain foods, beans,nuts, milk, unsweetened yogurt, cheese, cottage cheese, meats, fish, and eggs in addition to taking prenatal vitamins. They should eat foods that are high in protein; calcium; phosphorus; and vitamins A, C, and D. For snacks, suggest small amounts of non-cariogenic foods that are rich in protein, such as cheese.[22] If nausea prevents the patient from eating very much, suggest eating small quantities of healthy food throughout the day.[124,22]

2. Avoid Foods That Contains High Sugar

Reducing the number of foods that are high in sugar such as candy, desserts, and dried fruit is recommended.[124] Eating foods that are rich in fermentable carbohydrates or sugars, such as cookies, crackers, and chips, increases the risk of caries.

3. Drinks

Pregnant women should drink optimally fluoridated water, which the US Public Health Service has defined as 0.7 mg/L.[124] Alcoholic beverages should not be consumed during pregnancy.[124,20] Water or milk should be consumed in place of juice, fruit-flavored drinks, and carbonated beverages. The recommended daily fruit intake should be met by eating fruit rather than by drinking fruit juice.[22]

During meals, pregnant patients should reduce or eliminate drinking of the following:[22.124]

- Juice
- Soda; acids weaken tooth enamel
- Sports drinks
- Carbonated drinks

4. Folate

Adequate folate reduces the chance of cleft lip and palate.[22] Consumption of 0.4 mg of folic acid which is a synthetic version of folate at child bearing age is recommended. The US Public Health Service and Centers for Disease Control and Prevention in order to reduce the chance of birth defects when they become pregnant.[124]

Some foods are specifically fortified with folate or folic acid, and some foods naturally include folate, including:[124]

- Green leafy vegetables (Asparagus, broccoli, lettuce, spinach)
- Legumes (peas, lentils, and beans)
- Papaya, oranges, strawberries, cantaloupe, and bananas
- Tomato and orange juice

Anticipatory Dental Guidance

In order to help prepare the expectant mother for taking care of her infant anticipatory guidance should be provided. In addition, the expectant mother should be educated with what to expect and what steps she can take to make sure both herself and her infant will have good oral health.

Minimize Transmission of Cariogenic Bacteria

Educate the patient that saliva-sharing behavior such as the following may spread oral disease—including caries—to the infant:[22,113,24]

- Kissing the baby on the mouth.
- Sharing a spoon.
- Cleaning pacifier with your mouth.
- Licking your finger to wipe the baby's mouth.
- Allowing children to share toys, pacifiers, and other items that they can put in their mouths.
- Allowing older children to share straws, cups, or eating utensils, minimize cariogenic bacteria in people who are around the infant.

The main source of children's oral bacteria is her mothers oral bacteria. A mother with high levels of cariogenic bacteria is more likely to pass the cariogenic bacteria on to her infant.[22] Providing dental treatment to the mother and also to those around the infant will decrease the number of cariogenic bacteria that may be transferred to the infant.

The purpose of providing dental treatment is to improve the oral health of those around the infant, which in turn minimizes the transfer of cariogenic bacteria to the infant.[22] After pregnancy, encourage the woman to continue with dental care.[22]

5. Xylitol

One way to reduce cariogenic bacteria and improve oral health is to chew xylitol-containing gum or eating xylitol-containing products.

Maternal Use of Xylitol

Restorative dentistry by itself does not decrease the bacterial load sufficiently to prevent transmission to the infant—antibacterial treatment is also necessary. Antibacterial treatment may include fluoride, chlorhexidine, and xylitol usage.[22] Xylitol may be more effective than fluoride or chlorhexidine at reducing Streptococcus mutans levels in the mother and subsequently preventing caries in her children.[156] The anti-caries effect of xylitol appears to last for years.[156]

Xylitol Side Effects

Consuming 3 to 60 g of xylitol per day has resulted in patients experiencing abdominal distress and osmotic diarrhea.[141] Others have reported that osmotic diarrhea may occur when xylitol is consumed at four to five times that required for caries prevention,which is a total of 6 to 10 g of xylitol per day.[141]

Trimester	Recommendations
First trimester (1-13 weeks)	•Dental treatment should be limited to emergency and urgent needs. •If possible, avoid nitrous oxide •Periodontal treatment should be deferred. •Radiograghs should be limited for immediate treatment
Second trimester (14-26 weeks)	•It is the ideal time for dental treatment. •If topical and local anesthetic are inadequate for treatment nitrous oxide can be considered • It is the preferred time to perform periodontal treatment. This can include scaling, prophylaxis ,curettage and polishing •Routine radiographs should be avoided .
Third trimester (27 week-Delivery)	• In case the treatment cannot be postponed ,the patient should be treated by using left uterine displacement •If topical and local anesthetic are inadequate for treatment nitrous oxide can be considered •Periodontical treatment should be deffered. •Routine radiographs should be avoided .
Immediate postpartum (2-3 postpartum)	•Dental care is usally deferred. •Patient may be on prophylactic anticoagulative therapy as hypercoagulable state lasts for atleast 2-3 weks after birth , which increases the risk of bleeding. •The risk of pulmonary embolism is greater than during pregnancy

NOTE:

- Emergency and urgent dental treatment can be performed at any time of the pregnancy.
- Oral hygiene instructions should be provided to the patient constantly.
- Patient should be educated about the oral changes that occur during pregnancy
- Nutritional education along with anticipatory guidance should be provided

Guidance for Prenatal Care Health Professionals

In order to assess pregnant women's oral health, prenatal care health professionals may be the "first line" and they can provide referrals to oral health professionals and reinforce the preventive message.

Assess pregnant women's oral health status

Following are the steps to be followed during the initial prenatal evaluation:

- Take an oral health history.
- Check the mouth for problems such as swollen or bleeding gums, untreated dental decay, mucosal lesions, a sign of infection or trauma.
- Document your findings in the women's medical record.

Advise pregnant women about oral health care

- Reassure women that oral health care, including the use of radiographs, pain medication, and local anesthesia, is safe throughout pregnancy.
- If the last dental visit took place more than 6 months ago or if any oral health problems were identified during the assessment, the women is advised to schedule a dentist appointment as soon as possible. In case urgent care is needed one can write a formal referral to a dentist who maintains a cooperative relationship with the prenatal care health professional.
- **Encourage women to do take the following measures:**
    1. Seek oral health care
    2. Practice good oral hygiene
    3. Eat healthy foods
    4. Attend prenatal classes during pregnancy.
- In order to achieve and maintain optimal oral health the women should be counseled to follow recommendations given by the oral health professionals.

Work In Collaboration With Oral Health Professionals

- A relationship should be established with the oral health professionals in the community. A formal referral process should be developed as of which the oral health professional agrees to see the referred individual in a timely manner (e.g that day, the following day) in order to provide subsequent care.

Improve Health Services in the Community

- If beneficial provide a referral to a nutrition professional. Integrate oral health topics into prenatal classes. To provide care that is both culturally and linguistically appropriate. It is important to ensure that women understand the information that shared with them. Delaying necessary treatment for dental problems could result in significant risks to the mother and baby.

Get Oral Health Care

- It is important for the mother and baby to take care of your mouth while you are pregnant.
- It is safe throughout pregnancy to provide health care including the use of X-rays, pain medication, and local anesthesia.
- Before delivery get an oral health treatment as recommended by the professional.
- Schedule a dental appointment as soon as possible if you have any oral health problems or concerns or your last dental visit took place more than 6 months.
- Information like your due date will help the dental team provide the best care for you.

Practice Good Oral Hygiene

- Use fluoridated toothpaste twice a day. Replace your toothbrush every 3or 4 months, or more often if the bristles are frayed. Don't share your toothbrush with anyone. Clean between teeth daily with floss.
- Fluoridated, alcohol-free over-the-counter mouth rinse should be used every night
- Xylitol-containing gum or use other xylitol-containing products, such as mints, should be used which can help reduce bacteria that can cause tooth decay.
- A teaspoon of baking soda in a cup of water should be used to rinse your mouth after you vomit so as to stop acid from attacking your teeth.

Eat Healthy Foods

- One should eat a variety of healthy foods that includes: fruits, vegetables, whole-grain products (like cereals, bread, crackers), and dairy products such as cheese, milk, cottage cheese, or unsweetened yogurt. Some of the other good choices are meat, fish, chicken, eggs, beans, and nuts.
- Eating foods that are high in sugar like candy, cookies, cake, and dried fruit should be avoided, and high in sugar like juice, fruit-flavored drinks, or pop should be consumed in less quantity.
- The food that is chosen for snaking should be foods low in sugar such as fruits, vegetables, cheese, and unsweetened yogurt.
- Food labels should be read in order to find foods that are low in sugar.
- Small amounts of healthy food should be consumed throughout the day if dealing with nausea.
- Instead of juices, fruit-flavored drinks, or pop one should drink water or milk.
- Water should be drunk throughout the day, especially between meals and snacks.
- To reduce the risk of birth defects, get 600 mg of folic acid each day throughout your pregnancy. Take a dietary supplement of folic acid and eat food high in folate and foods fortified with folic acid.

Practice Other Healthy Behaviors

- Attends prenatal classes.
- Usage of tobacco products and recreational drugs should be stopped. Also one should also avoid secondhand smoke.
- Stop any consumption of alcoholic beverages.

COVID-19 and Pregnancy

According to numerous studies all around the world it has been deduced that pregnant women are not more likely to get COVID19 than other healthy adults. About 2/3rd of the pregnant women do not show any COVID-19 symptoms, and rest of the pregnant women who exhibit symptoms only have mild cold or flu-like symptoms. however the pregnant women are at increased risk of becoming severely unwell if they catch COVID-19 if they are unvaccinated or not fully vaccinated, which can lead to premature birth of the baby and admission to intensive care.[157]

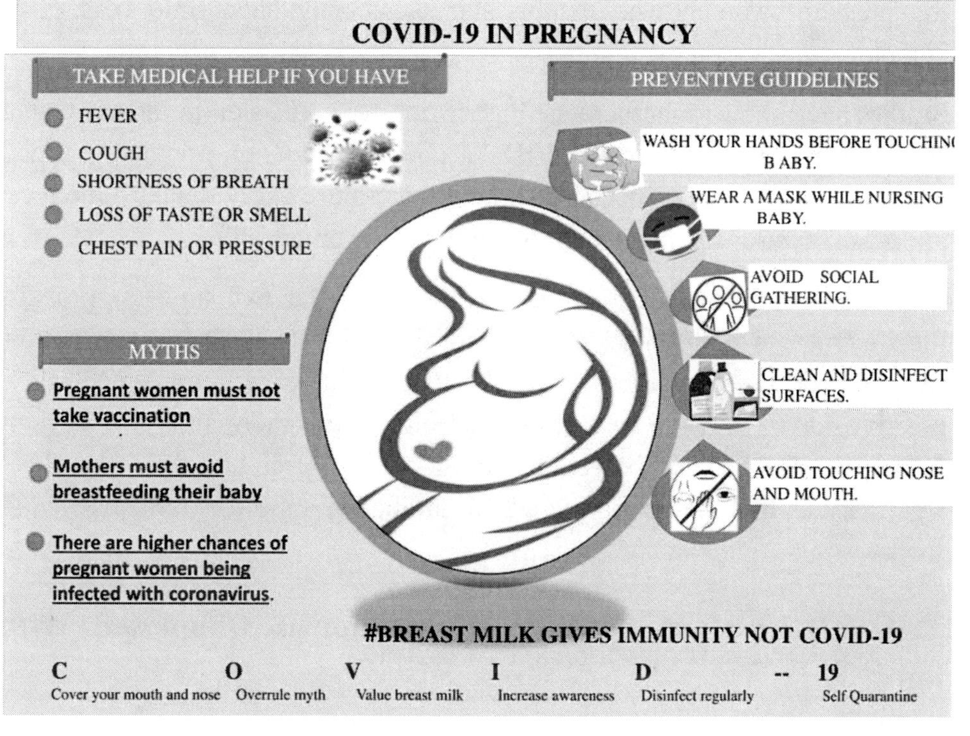

Key advice for pregnant women:

- It is strongly recommended to take two doses of the COVID 19 vaccine and the booster dose at any stage of pregnancy. It is the safest and most effective way of protecting you and your baby from COVID-19 infection
- Pregnant women should be prioritize for the booster vaccination.
- In order to stay safe and to prevent the spread of COVID 19 pregnant women should follow government guidance:

- Stay active with regular exercise, a healthy balanced diet, and folic acid and vitamin D supplementation so as to support a healthy pregnancy.
- Dont miss any of the pregnancy scans and antenatal appointments unless you are advised otherwise.
- If you have concerns regarding the well-being of yourself or your unborn baby you should contact your maternity team.

Effect that COVID-19 have on pregnant women:

- The Current proofs from the UK indicates that the pregnant women aren't more likely to get COVID-19 than any other healthy adults, however the pregnant women are at increased risk of becoming severely unwell if they catch COVID-19 if they are unvaccinated or not fully vaccinated, which can lead to admission to intensive care and premature birth of the baby. About 2/3rd of the pregnant women do not show any COVID-19 symptoms ie. Are asymptomatic, and rest of the pregnant women who exhibit symptoms only have mild cold or flu-like symptoms.
- Studies have shown that there are higher rates of admission to intensive care units for pregnant women with COVID-19 compared to non-pregnant women with COVID-19, this may be because clinicians are more likely to take a more cautious approach towards the pregnant women when a woman is pregnant.
- In pregnant ladies with signs of COVID-19, it's far two times as probable that their infant can be born early, exposing the infant to the danger of prematurity. Several worldwide research have also found that pregnant women who tested positive for COVID-19 at the time of birth were more likely to develop pre-eclampsia, more likely to need an emergency c-section and their risk of stillbirth was twice as high, although the actual number of stillbirths remains significantly low.

Effect COVID-19 Have on Baby If Mother is Diagnosed With the Infection

Current evidence indicates that if a pregnant women is diagnosed with COVID19 it is is unlikely to cause problems with the baby's development.

There is likewise no proof to signify that COVID-19 infection in early pregnancy increases the chance of a miscarriage.

Vertical transmission of COVID19 from a woman to her baby during pregnancy or childbirth seems to be uncommon. The mode of birth i.e. vaginal birth or caesarean does not determine whether or not the newborn gets COVID19. In most of the reported cases of new-born babies remained well after developing COVID-19 very soon after birth.

Any concerns or questions should be discussed with your local maternity unit. You can also check on arrangements for all scheduled and future appointments.

Conclusion

In order to provide dental treatment to a pregnant patient, additional consideration may be needed. for routine dental treatment for a healthy pregnant woman, there are circumstances and treatment options whereas consult with the patient's prenatal care provider is required and is recommended.[22,113,117,120,124] In order to establish a trusting relationship with the patient for future care, the patient should still be educated even if the treatment is not available.

Dental care should not be deferred for the absolute reason of pregnancy. Oral care during pregnancy involves the contribution of patients, dental professionals, and physicians and is very important. Patients during pregnancies must be educated about the following:

a) Importance of maintaining good oral hygiene.

b) Expected changes in the oral cavity.

c) Routine dental visits.

In order to provide the best level of patient care referral and consultation to the patient's gynecologist or physician should be considered. There should be limited use of drug therapy and should be carried out carefully. Radiotherapy and elective surgery should be avoided. For time management the female patients of childbearing age or expecting females should be screened for caries and oral diseases.[158]

Changes in dental anxiety may require modification regarding what is included in the treatment plan and when treatment will be completed as well as extra reassurance to the patient and the presentation of additional information when obtaining informed consent. Variations in her vital signs may either be normal pregnancy-related physiologic changes or may indicate the presence of pathology that should be brought to the attention of the patient's prenatal care provider.

Pregnancy-related oral problems can develop and may require treatments. Some of the pregnancy-related problems may include:

- Perimylolysis (enamel erosion/decalcification)
- Pregnancy gingivitis
- Gingival hyperplasia
- Pyogenic granuloma
- Salivary changes.

In order to minimize the adverse impact that can be caused due to possible decreased circulation for both the expectant mother and unborn baby, the patient positioning should be modified from supine to LUD as the pregnancy progresses. There are many pregnancy-related medical conditions that may initially need management by dental professionals. These may include: hypoglycemia(from gestational diabetes), nosebleeds, Braxton-Hicks contractions (false labor), hyperventilation, dyspnea (shortness of breath), and morning sickness. The expectant mother should be educated by providing her with nutritional counseling, oral hygiene instruction, and anticipatory guidance.

Reference

1. Patil S, Thakur R, Paul ST, Gadicherla P. Oral healthcoalition: knowledge, attitude, practice behaviours among gynaecologistsand dental practitioners. J Int Oral Health, 2013;5:8–15.
2. Tracy MDellinger H. Mark Livingston. Pregnancy: Physiological changes and considerations for dental patients. Dent Clin N Am, 2006;50:677-97
3. American Academy on Pediatric Dentistry Council on Clinical Affairs Committee on the adolescent. Guidelines on oral health care for the pregnant adolescent. Pediatr Dent, 2008-2009;30:102-06.
4. Stalp S, Zuhrt R. Dental caries and pregnancy. Stomatol DDR,1979; 29: 481- 4.
5. Gaffield ML, Gilbert BJ, Malvitz DM, Romaguera R. Oral health duringpregnancy: an analysis of information collected by the pregnancy risk assessmentmonitoring system. J Am Dent Assoc, 2001;132: 1009-16.
6. StefanacSJ, Nesbit SP. Treatment planning in Dentistry.St Louis:Elsevier; 2001.
7. Wasylko L, Matsui D, Dykxhoorn SM, Rieder MJ, Weinberg S. A review ofcommon dental treatments during pregnancy: implications for patients and dentalpersonnel. J Can Dent Assoc 1998; 64: 434-9.
8. Suresh L, Radfar L. Pregnancy and lactation. Oral Surg Oral Med Oral PatholOral Radiol Endod. 2004;97:672-82.
9. Turner M, Aziz SR. Management of the pregnant oral and maxillofacial surgery patient. J Oral Maxillofac Surg, 2002;60:1479–88.
10. Mabie WC, Di Sessa TG, Crocker LG, et al. A longitudinalstudy of cardiac output in normal human pregnancy. Am J ObstetGynecol, 1994;170:849–56.
11. LeeW.Cardiorespiratory alterations during normal pregnancy. Crit Care Clin,1991;7:763-75
12. .Hunter S, Robson SC. Adaptation of the maternal heart in pregnancy. Br Heart J,1992;99:540–3.
13. Chu ZM, Beilin LJ. Mechanisms of vasodilation in pregnancy: studies of the role of prostaglandins and nitric oxide in changes of vascular reactivity in the in situ blood perfused mesentery of pregnant rats. Br J Pharmacol, 1993;109:322–9.
14. Theunissen IM, Parer JT. Fluid and electrolytes in pregnancy. Clin Obstet Gynecol, 1994;37:3–15.

15. Duvekot JJ, Peeters LL. Maternal cardiovascular hemodynamic adaptation to pregnancy. ObstetGynecolSurv, 1994;49:S1–14.

16. Baron WM, Lindheimer MD. Medical disorders during pregnancy. 2nd ed. St Louis: Mosby; 1995.

17. Thornburg KL, Jacobson SL, Giraud GD. Hemodynamic changes in pregnancy.SeminPerinatol, 2000;24:11–4.

18. Clark SL, Cotton DB, Lee W. Central hemodynamic assessment of normal term pregnancy. Am J ObstetGynecol, 1989;161:1439–42.

19. Clapp JF, Capeless E. Cardiovascular function before, during, and after the first and subsequent pregnancies. Am J Cardiol, 1997;80:1469–73.

20. Hilgers KK, Douglass J, Mathieu GP. Adolescent pregnancy: A review of dental treatment guidelines. Pediatr Dent, 2003;25:459–467.

21. Fayans EP, Stuart HR, Carsten D, Ly Q, Kim H. Local anesthetic use in the pregnant and postpartum patient. Dent Clin North Am, 2010;54:697–713.

22. California Dental Association Foundation, American College of Obstetricians and Gynecologists, District IX. Oral health during pregnancy and early childhood: Evidence-based guidelines for health professionals. J Calif Dent Assoc, 2010;38:391–403.

23. The American College of Obstetricians and Gynecologists. Definition of Term Pregnancy. Committee Opinion Number 579. http://www.acog.org//media/Committee-Opinions/Committee-on-Obstetric-Practice. Last Accessed on 28 November 2019.

24. Stevens J, Iida H, Ingersoll G. Implementing an oral health program in a group prenatal practice. JObstetGynecol Neonatal Nurs, 2007;36:581–591.

25. American Academy of Pediatric Dentistry. Guideline on fluoride therapy. Pediatr Dent, 2013;35:E165–E168

26. Jeejeebhoy FM, Zelop CM, Lipman S, et al. Cardiac arrest in pregnancy: A scientific statement from the American Heart Association. JCirculation, 2015;132:1747–1773.

27. Campbell TA, Sanson TG. Cardiac arrest and pregnancy. J Emerg Trauma Shock, 2009;2:34–42.

28. Goodwin AP, Pearce AJ. The human wedge. A manoeuvre to relieve aortocaval compression during resuscitation in late pregnancy. Anaesthesia, 1992;47:433–434

29. Rees GA, Willis BA. Resuscitation in late pregnancy. J Anaesthesia,1988;43:347–349.

30. Garcia-Rio F, Pino JM, Gomez L, et al. Regulation of breathing and perception of dyspnea in healthy pregnant women. J Chest, 1996;110:446–53.

31. McAuliffe F, Kametas N, Costello J, et al. Respiratory function in singleton and twin pregnancy. BJOG, 2002;109:765–9.

32. Skatrud JB, Dempsey JA, Kaiser DG. Ventilatory response to medroxyprogesterone acetate in normal subjects. J ApplPhysiol Respir Environ Exerc Physiol, 1978;44:393–44.

33. Camann WR, Ostheimer GW. Physiological adaptations during pregnancy. Int Anesthesiol Clin,1990; 28:2.

34. Hankins GDV, Clark SL, Harvey CJ. Third-trimester arterial blood gas and acid base values in normal pregnancy at moderate altitude. Obstet Gynecol,1996;88:347.

35. Awe RJ, Nicotra MB, Newsom TD. Arterial oxygenation and alveolar-arterial gradients in term pregnancy. ObstetGynecol, 1979;53:182.

36. Barron WM.Medical evaluation of the pregnant patient requiring nonobstetric surgery. Clin Perinatol, 1985;12:481–96.

37. Branch DW. Physiologic adaptations of pregnancy. Am J Reprod Immunol, 1992;28:120–2.

38. Hamaoui E, Hamaoui M. Nutritional assessment and support during pregnancy. Gastroenterol Clin North Am, 2003;32:59–121.

39. NIH Consensus Development Congress. Prevention of venous thrombosis and pulmonary embolism. JAMA, 1986;256:744–9.

40. Letsky EA, DeSwiet M. Thromboembolism in pregnancy and its management. Br J Haematol, 1984;57:543–52.

41. Rutherford SE, Phelan JP. Thromboembolic disease in pregnancy. Clin Perinatol, 1988;13:719–39.

42. Barbour L. Current concepts of anticoagulant therapy in pregnancy. ObstetGynecol Clin North Am, 1997;28:499–521.

43. Hunt MG, Martin JN, Martin RW. Perinatal aspects of abdominal surgery for nonobstetric disease. Am J Perinatol, 1989;6:412–7.

44. Hanly JG. Antiphospholipid syndrome: an overview. CMAJ,2003;24(168):1675–82.

45. Sherman P, Flaxman SM. Nausea and vomiting of pregnancy in an evolutionary perspective. Am J Obstet Gynecol, 2002;185:s190–7.

46. Calhoun BC. Gastrointestinal disorders in pregnancy. ObstetGynecol Clin North Am, 1992;4:733–44.

47. Christofides ND, Ghatei MA, Bloom SR. Decreased plasma motilin concentrations in pregnancy. Br Med J, 1982;285:1453.

48. Ch'ng CL, Morgan M, Hainsworth I, et al. Prospective study of liver dysfunction in Southwest Wales. J Gut, 2002;51:876–80.

49. Martin C, Varner MW. Physiologic changes in pregnancy: surgical implications. Clin Obstet Gynecol, 1994;37:241–55.

50. Koch KL, Frissora CL. Nausea and vomiting during pregnancy. Gastroenterol Clin North Am, 2003;32(1):201–34.

51. Koch KL. Gastrointestinal factors in nausea and vomiting of pregnancy. Am J ObstetGynecol, 2002;186(5 Suppl): S198–203.

52. Crawford JS, Oppit LJ. A survey of anesthetic services to obstetrics in the Birmingham Hospital. Reg Anesth, 1976;31:56–9.

53. Bond VK, Stoelting RK, Gupta CD. Pulmonary aspiration syndrome after inhalation of gastric fluid containing antacids. Anesthesiology, 1979;51:452–3.

54. Gibbs CP, Banner TC. Effectiveness of Bicitra as a preoperative antacid. Anesthesiology, 1984;61:97–9.

55. Gibbs CP, Spohr L, Shmidt D. The effectiveness of sodium citrate as an antacid. Anesthesiology, 1982;57:44–6.

56. Hodgkinson R, Glassenberg R, Joyce TH III. Comparison of cimetidine with antacid for safety and effectiveness in reducing gastric acidity before elective cesarean section. Anesthesiology,1983;59: 86–90.

57. Yau G, Kan AF, Gin T. A comparison of omeprazole and ranitidine for prophylaxis against aspiration pneumonitis in emergency caesarean section. Anaesthesia, 1992;47:101.

58. Dafnis E, Sabatini S. The effect of pregnancy on renal function: physiology and pathophysiology.AmJ Med Sci, 1992;303:184–205.

59. Davidson JM, Renal disorders in pregnancy.CurrOpinObstet Gynecol, 2001;13:109-14

60. Davidson JM, Shiells EA, Philips PR, et al. Serial evaluation of vasopressin release and thirst in human pregnancy: role of human chorionic gonadotropin in the osmoregulatory changes of gestation. J Clin Invest, 1988;81:798–806.

61. Diokno AC, Compton A, Seski J. Urologic evaluation of urinary tract infection in pregnancy. J Reprod Med, 1986;31:23–6.

62. Mikhail MS, Anyaegbunam A. Lower urinary tract dysfunction in pregnancy: a review. ObstetGynecol Surv, 1995;50:675–83.

63. Soory M. Hormonal factors in periodontal disease. Dent Update, 2000; 27:380-83.

64. Gajendra S, Kumar JV.Oral health and pregnancy: A review. N Y State Dent J, 2004;70:40-44.

65. Yuan K, Wing LY, Lin MT. Pathogenetic roles of angiogenic factors in pyogenic granulomas in pregnancy are modulated by female sex hormones. J Periodontol, 2002;73:701-08.

66. Kim AJ, Lo AJ, Pullin DA, Thornton-Johnson DS, Karimbux NY. Scaling and root planing treatment for periodontitis to reduce preterm birth and low birth weight: A systematic review andmeta-analysis of randomized controlled trials. J Periodontol, 2012;83:1508–1519.

67. Richter JE. Gastroesophageal reflux disease during pregnancy. Gastroenterol Clin N Am.2003; 32:235-61.

68. Agueda A, Echeverria A, Manau C. Association between periodontitis in pregnancy and preterm or low birth weight: Review of the literature. Med Oral Patol Cir Bucal, 2008;13:E609-15.

69. Chaveli Lopez B, Sarrion Perez MG, Jimenez Soriano Y. Dental considerations in pregnancy and menopause. J Clin Exp Dent, 2011;3(2):e135-44.

70. Kandan PM, Menaga V, Kumar RRR, Oral health in pregnancy. J PakMed, 2011;61:1009-14.

71. Sacco G, Carmagnola D, Abati S, Luglio PF et al. Periodotal disease and preterm birth relationship. Minerva Stomatol, 2008;57:233-46, 246-50.

72. Lee RV. Medical care of the pregnant patient. Philadelphia: ACP-ASIM;2000.

73. Page EW, Page EP. Leg cramps in pregnancy. Obstet Gynecol, 1953;1:94–100

74. Monga M. Maternal–fetal medicine: principles and practice. Philadelphia: W.B. Saunders;2004.

75. Berg G, Hammar M, Moller-Nielsen J. Low back pain during pregnancy. Obstet Gynecol, 1988:71–5.

76. Cogen RB.Special andmedically compromised patients in dentistry: PSG Publishing; 1989.

77. Mason ED.Medical care of the pregnant patient. Philadelphia: ACP-ASIM ;2000.

78. Gillogley KM, Evens AT, Hansen RL. The impact of cocaine, amphetamine, and opiate use detected by universal intrapartum screening. Am J ObstetGynecol, 1990;163:1535–42.

79. Statewide prevalence of illicit drug use by pregnant womendRhode Island. Morb MortalWkly Rep, 1990;39:354–5.

80. Simpson WJ. A preliminary report on cigarette smoking and the incidence of prematurity. Am J Obstet Gynecol,1957;73:808.]

81. Andres RL. Maternal–fetalmedicine: principles and practice. Philadelphia: W.B. Saunders; 2004.

82. LattsLM. Medical care of the pregnant patient. Philadelphia: ACP-ASIM;2000.

83. Manning FA, Feyerabend C. Cigarette smoking and fetal breathing movements. Br J Obstet Gynaecol, 1976;83:262.

84. Longo LD, Ching KS. Placental diffusing capacity for carbon monoxide and oxygen inunanesthetized sheep. J Appl Physiol, 1977;43:885.

85. Klesges LM, Johnson KC, Ward KD. Smoking cessation in pregnant women. ObstetGynecol Clin North Am, 2001;28:26

86. Melvin C, Dolan MP, Windsor RA. Recommended cessation counseling for pregnantwomen who smoke: a review of the evidence. Tob Control, 2000;9:80.

87. Mullen P. Maternal smoking during pregnancy and evidence-based intervention topromote cessation. Prim Care, 1999;26:578.

88. Benowitz NL, Dempsey DA, Goldenberg RL. The use of pharmacotherapies for smokingcessation during pregnancy. Tob Control, 2000;9(3):91.

89. Nagy. Intensive outpatient treatment for alcohol and other drug abuse: United States Department of Health and Human Services; 1994.

90. Gehshan S. Missed opportunities for intervening in the lives of pregnant women addicted to alcohol or other drugs. Journal of American Medical Women Association, 1995;50:160–3.

91. Coles CD. Impact of prenatal alcohol exposure on the newborn and the child. Clin ObstetGynecol, 1993;36:255.

92. Clarren SK. Recognition of fetal alcohol syndrome. JAMA, 1981;245:2436–9.

93. Ritchie J, Greene N. Local anesthetics. Thepharmacological basis of therapeutics. New York: Macmillan;1985.

94. Woods JR, Plessinger MA, Clark KE. Effect of cocaine on uterine blood flow and fetal oxygenation. JAMA, 1987;257:957–61.

95. Briggs GG, Freeman RK, Yaffe SJ. Drugs in pregnancy and lactation. LWW,2005;7:168–71,362–77,714–7, 1249–51.

96. Mittleman RE, Corofino JC, Hearn WL. Tissue distribution of cocaine in a pregnantwoman. J ForensicSci, 1989;34:481–6.

97. Hurd WW, Betz AL, Dombrowski MP, et al. Cocaine augments contractility of the pregnant human uterus by both adrenergic and non-adrenergic mechanisms. Am J Obstet Gynecol, 1998;178:1077–81.

98. Stalp S, Zuhrt R. Dental caries and pregnancy. Stomatol DDR,1979; 29: 481- 4.

99. U.S. Depa. of Health and Human Services, National Instituteof Dental and Craniofacial Research. Oral Health in America: A Report of the Surgeon General.

NIH publication no. 00-4713. Rockville, Md.: U.S. Public Health Service, Dept. of Health and Human Services; 2000.

100. Sills ES, Zegarelli DJ, Hoschander MM, Strider WE. Clinical diagnosis and management of hormonally responsive oral pregnancy tumour (pyogenic granuloma). J Reprod Med,1996; 41: 467-70.

101. Kumar J, Samelson R. Oral health care during pregnancy and early childhood: practice guidelines. NewYork, NY: New York State Department of Health, 2006.

102. American Academy of Periodontology. Periodontal (gum) diseases.http://www.perio.org/consumer/2a. html. Last Accessed on August 1, 2019.

103. Goepfert AR, Jeffcoat MK, Andrews WW, et al. Periodontal disease and upper genital tract inflammation in early spontaneous preterm birth. Obstet Gyneco. 2004;104(4):777-783.

104. Offenbacher S, Lieff S, Boggess KA, et al. Maternal periodontitis and prematurity. Part I: obstetric outcome of prematurity and growth restriction. Ann Periodontol, 2001;6(1):164-174.

105. Task Force on Periodontal Treatment of Pregnant Women, American Academy of Periodontology. American Academy of Periodontology statement regarding periodontal management of the pregnant patient. J Periodontol, 2004;75(3):495.

106. American Academy of Pediatric Dentistry. Guideline on Oral Health Care for the Pregnant Adolescent. http://www.aapd.org/media/Policies_Guidelines/G_Pregnancy.pdf. Last Accessed on 29 August 2019.

107. Olsen RN, Dunsmoor-Su R, Capurro D, McMahon K, Gravett MG. Correlation between spontaneous preterm birth and mid-trimester maternal serium estriol. J MaternFetal Neonatal Med, 2014;27:376–380.

108. Priya B, Mustafa MD, Guleria K, Vaid NB, Banerjee BD, Ahmed RS. Salivary progesterone as a biochemical marker to predict early preterm birth in asymptomatic high-risk women. BJOG, 2013;120:1003–1011.

109. US Department of Health and Human Services, Food and Drug Administration. Reviewer Guidance: Evaluating the Risks of Drug Exposure in Human Pregnancies. https://www.fda.gov/downloads/Drugs/.../Guidances/ucm071645.pdf. Last Accessed on 28 july 2019.

110. Sader TW. Langman's Medical Embryology. ed 8. Baltimore: Lippincott Williams & Wilkins;2000.

111. Donaldson M, Goodchild JH. Pregnancy, breast-feeding and drugs used in dentistry. J Am Dent Assoc, 2012;143:858–871.

112. Niessen LC. The ADA Practical Guide to Patients with Medical Conditions. Ames, Iowa: Wiley-Blackwell;2012.

113. New York State Department of Health. Oral Health Care During Pregnancy and Early Childhood: Practice Guidelines. https://www.health.ny.gov/publications/0824.pdf.Last Accessed on 10 october 2019.

114. Sonis ST, Fazio RC, Fang LST. Principles and Practice of Oral Medicine.ed 2. Philadelphia: Saunders;1995.

115. Flynn TR, Susarla SM. Oral and maxillofacial surgery for the pregnant patient. Oral Maxillofac Surg Clin North Am, 2007;19:207–221.

116. Hashim and Akbar, Gynecologists knoeledge regarding periodontal disease and pregnancy outcome. Jispcd, 2018;4:166-72.

117. Steinberg BJ, Hilton IV, Iada H, Samelson R. Oral health and dental care during pregnancy. Dent Clin North Am, 2013;57:195–210.

118. US Food and Drug Administration. FDA Pregnancy and Lactation Labeling (Drugs) FinalRule.http://www.fda.gov/Drugs/DevelopmentApprovalProcess/DevelopmentResources/Labeling/ucm093307.htm. Last Accessed on 25 June 2019.

119. Ritter AV, Southerland JH. Pregnancy and oral health. J EsthetRestor Dent, 2007;19:373–374.

120. Achtari MD, Georgakopoulou EA, Afentoulide N. Dental care throughout pregnancy: What a dentist must know. J Oral Health Dent Manag, 2012;11:169–176.

121. Wong D, Cheng A, Kunchur R, Lam S, Sambrook PJ, Goss AN. Management of severe odontogenic infections in pregnancy. Aust Dent J, 2012;57:498–503.

122. Moore PA. Selecting drugs for the pregnant dental patient. J Am Dent Assoc, 1998;129:1281–1286.

123. Cengiz SB The pregnant patient: Considerations for dental management and drug use. Quintessence Int, 2007;38:e133–e142.

124. Oral Health Care During Pregnancy Expert Workgroup. Oral health care during pregnancy: A national consensus statement. Washington, DC: National Maternal and Child Oral Health Resource Center, 2012.

125. Naseem M, Khurshid Z, Hammad KA, Niazi F, Zohaib S, Zafar et al.Oral health challenges in pregnant women:Recommendations for dental care professionals. The Saudi J Dent Res, 2016;7:138-46.

126. American Dental Association. Dental Radiographic Examinations: Recommendations for Patient Selection and Limiting Radiation Exposure. http://www.ada.org/~/media/ADA/Member%20. Last assesd on 10 Dec 2010.

127. Nguyen CP, Goodman LH. Fetal risk in diagnostic radiology. Semin Ultrasound CT MR, 2012;33:4–10.

128. Luglie PF, Campus G, Chessa G, et al. Effect of amalgam fillings on the mercury concentration in human amniotic fluid. Arch Gynecol Obstet, 2005;271:138–142.

129. Watson GE, Lynch M, Myers GJ, et al. Prenatal exposure to dental amalgam. Evidence from the Sychelles Child Development Study main cohort. J Am Dent Assoc, 2011;142:1283–1294.

130. American Dental Association. Dental Amalgam: What Others Say. www.ada.org.

131. Chen L, Suh BI. Bisphenol A in dental materials: A review. JSM Dent,2013;1:1004.

132. Fischer D. Ultradent's Vigilance with BPA. https://www.ultradent.com/zh-cn/Dental-Products/Prevent-Hygiene/Pit-and-Fissure-Sealants/UltraSeal-XT-hydro-hydrophilic-sealant/Documents/BPA Letter from Dr. Fischer_Website.pdf. Last Accessed on 22 August 2019.

133. Moore PA. Selecting drugs for the pregnant dental patient. J Am Dent Assoc, 1998;129:1281–1286.

134. Silk H, DouglassAB, Douglass JM,SilkL, Oral health during pregnancy. Am Fam Physican, 2008;77(8):1139-44.

135. Buprofen: Ibuprofen Tablet, Film Coated [package insert]. Bachepalli, India: Dr. Reddy's Laboratories Limited, 2007.

136. Wynn RL, Meiller TF, Crossley HL (eds). Drug Information Handbook for Dentistry, ed 23. Hudson, OH: Lexi-Comp, 2018.

137. Lodi KB, Carvalho LF, Koga-Ito CY, Carvalho VA, Rocha RF. Rational use of antimicrobials in dentistry during pregnancy. Med Oral Patol Oral Cir Bucal, 2009;14:E15–E19.

138. Aldred KJ, Kerns RJ, Osheroff N. Mechanism of quinolone action and resistance. Biochemistry, 2014;53:1565–1574.

139. Cipro [package insert]. West Haven, CT: Bayer, 2004.

140. Penicillin V Potassium [package insert]. Fort Lee, NJ: Dava Pharmaceuticals, 2011.

141. Ly KA, Milgrom P, Rothen M. Xylitol, sweeteners, and dental caries. Pediatr Dent,2006;28:154–163.

142. Jacobsen PL. The Little Dental Drug Booklet: Handbook of Commonly Used Dental Medicationsed 20, Hudson,OH: Lexicomp; 2013.

143. Dicloxacillin Sodium: Dicloxacillin Sodium Capsule [package insert]. Sellersville, PA: Teva Pharmaceuticals, 2011.

144. Clindamycin Hydrochloride: Clindamycin Hydrochloride Capsule [package insert]. Concord, NC:McKesson Corporation; 2009.

145. Hemalatha VT, ManigandanT, Amudhan A. Pregnancyand oral care. JCDR, 2013;7(5):948-53.

146. Malamed SF. Handbook of Local Anesthesia. ed 6, St Louis: Elsevier; 2013.

147. Jacobsen RB, Borche JE, Bindslev-Jensen C. Hypersensitivity to local anaesthetics. Allergy, 2005;60:262–264.

148. Lidocaine Hydrochloride: Lidocaine Hydrochloride Anhydrous Solution [package insert]. Amityville, NY: Hi-Tech Pharmacal, 2011.

149. Cetacaine Topical Anesthetic: Benzocaine, Butamben, and Tetracaine Hydrochloride Gel [packageinsert]. Pennsauken, NJ: Cetylite Industries, 2010.

150. Lidocaine: Lidocaine Ointment [package insert]. Hawthorne, NY: Taro Pharmaceuticals, 2005.

151. Oraqix (Lidocaine and Prilocaine Periodontal Gel) 2.5% / 2.5% [package insert]. York, PA: Dentsply Pharmaceutical, 2010.

152. Octocaine (Lidocaine Hydrochloride and Epinephrine Injection, USP) [package insert].Cambridge, Canada: Novocol Pharmaceutical of Canada, 2007.

153. Toxicology Data Network. Tetracaine. http://toxnet.nlm.nih.gov/cgi-bin/sis/search2/r?dbs+lactmed:@. Last Accessed on 30 July 2019.

154. VivacaineBupivicaine HCl 0.5% and Epinephrine 1:200,000 Injection (as Bitartrate) [package insert].Cambridge, Canada: Novocol Pharmaceutical of Canada, 2009.

155. American Dental Association. Oral Health Topics: Toothpastes. http://www.ada.org/en/member-center/oral-health-topics/toothpastes.Last Accessedon 22 July 2019.

156. American Academy on Pediatric Dentistry. Policy on the Use of Xylitol. http://www.aapd.org/media/Policies_Guidelines/P_Xylitol.pdf. Last Accessed on 22 September 2019.

157. https://www.cdc.gov/coronavirus/2019-ncov/need-extra-precautions/pregnant-people.html.

158. Zambrano LD, Ellington S, Strid P, et al. Update: Characteristics of Symptomatic Women of Reproductive Age with Laboratory-Confirmed SARS-CoV-2 Infection by Pregnancy Status — United States, January 22–October 3, 2020. MMWR Morb Mortal Wkly Rep 2020;69:1641–1647. DOI: 10.15585/mmwr.mm6944e3.